SHERYL FEUTZ-HARTER

W9-BMW-424

Legal &
Ethical
Standards
FOR NURSES

PESi HealthCare

**For information on this and other PESI HealthCare manuals
and audiocassettes, please call**

800-843-7763

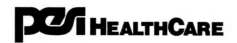

ACKNOWLEDGEMENTS

This book is possible only because of dear and supportive friends and colleagues, and my wonderful son, Evan, an extremely understanding and flexible 11-year-old. Most importantly, it's the result of the expert qualities, endless energy, and special efforts of my secretary at Shughart Thomson & Kilroy, P.C., Shana Lee Koelling, for and to whom I am extremely grateful and blessed. Extra special thanks also to Jennifer Marsh, Esq., Jim Coulter, Nurse Paralegal/Consultant, and Betty Sola, Librarian Extraordinaire!

I dedicate this book to my late husband, Evan's dad, and my best friend, Tim Harter, to whom I am indebted for the completeness of my life and my sense of humor.

About the Author

Sheryl Feutz-Harter is Of Counsel with the law firm of Shughart Thomson & Kilroy, in its Kansas City, Missouri office where she has practiced law since 1986. Her law practice focuses on health care law, professional licensure actions, and corporate compliance for health care providers. Sheryl is also Vice President and General Counsel/Compliance and Security Officer for New Directions Behavioral Health in Shawnee Mission, Kansas. Sheryl is a registered nurse, having received her B.S.N. degree from the University of Missouri-Columbia and her M.S.N. degree in community health nursing from the University of Alabama—Birmingham. She received her law degree from Loyola Law School in Los Angeles, California. Sheryl is on the Adjunct Faculty of the University of Missouri—Columbia School of Nursing where she regularly teaches classes on legal issues to nursing students. She also frequently gives presentations on health care legal issues throughout the country. Sheryl is a member of many local, state, and national legal and nursing organizations, and is involved in various community activities.

TABLE OF CONTENTS

PREFACE

Nursing began as women providing nurturing to the ill and injured. The necessary skills were caring, empathy, and compassion. While these skills remain essential ingredients for effective nursing care, they now only complement other critical skills such as scientific knowledge, technical performance, and teaching ability. A sound understanding of ethical principles and the legal system, and how they impact nurses and patients is also required.

My continuing commitment to patients and to nurses resulted in this book. As health care delivery systems, professional responsibilities, and scientific advances evolve, so must the resources and critical thinking about the legal and ethical standards applicable for nurses today. Yet this book is not exhaustive of *all* legal and ethical considerations that are applicable, nor does it consider many other important factors specific to each patient situation, such as religious, social, moral, and financial issues. Additionally, each State has laws that will impact actions, and those are constantly changing.

THIS BOOK DOES NOT REPLACE SEEKING LEGAL ADVICE FOR SPECIFIC FACT SITUATIONS.

—S. F. H.
November 2003

CHAPTER 1

Introduction

Guess what? Nurses make errors! Nurses are human beings, and "human beings, in all lines of work, make errors."[1] So, how do nurses handle this stark realization? I wish I had the solution to create a perfect "system" for health care; if I did, I'd write that book instead of this one!

First as a nurse, and now as an attorney, I have focused my professional life on improving the quality of care and quality of life of patients by focusing on the health care system and providers who impact those qualities. While I see myself as an optimistic person, I don't believe there will ever be a "perfect" health care system. However, I believe there are multiple ways that the health care system and the care provided by health care providers, especially nurses, can be improved. Many of the health care deficiencies result from lacking knowledge of laws that protect patients. These "laws" consist of statutes, regulations, standards of care, common law, ethical codes, policies, clinical practice guidelines, research, just to name a few. Since I find it challenging to keep abreast of all of these laws (and I don't even have to stay current with nursing and medical practices!), this is my attempt to help you at least know where to begin to become knowledgeable about laws that will enable you to provide a higher quality of nursing care. While these are exciting and challenging times for nurses clinically, they are equally challenging legally.

But how do I approach discussing "health care law" as it impacts nurses when there is no clear description of what "health care law" includes. The consensus is that there are no consistent descriptive terms for "health care law," which is sometimes referred to as "law and medicine," "law and nursing," "med-

---

1 Institute of Medicine, Committee on Quality of Healthcare in America. *To Err is Human: Building a Safer Health System.* (2000).

ical jurisprudence," "health risk management." In actuality, health care law is "largely a creature of happenstance . . . and consists of disparate areas of law and regulation that happen to apply to doctors, hospitals, and health insurers . . . ."[2] The analogy Hall used in his article is comparing nurses with horses, referencing the following quote: "Lots of cases deal with sales of horses; others deal with people kicked by horses; still more deal with the licensing and racing of horses, or with the care veterinarians give to horses, or with prizes at horse shows. Any effort to collect these strands into a course on "The Law of the Horse" is doomed to be shallow and misunifying principles.[3] This certainly reflects the complexity of the laws that affect nurses.

Perhaps a better term for "health care law" is "therapeutic jurisprudence," which was first conceived by David Wexler and Bruce Winick to identify what approach the law should take in reference to patients with behavioral health disorders.[4] Does it consider the effect it produces on relationships between nurses and patients? The premise is the person and dignity of each person must be respected and laws are used to benefit the health and well-being of patients. The effect of the laws is to achieve therapeutic goals that are in the best interest of these patients. Approaching health care law from a therapeutic prospective is certainly consistent with the roles and goals of nurses.

And what is critical to achieving therapeutic health care goals? Trust, the integrity of the relationship between the nurse and the patient and between nurses and other health care providers. It is the basis for the patient believing in the confidentiality of communications with nurses and the willingness to expose ones innermost vulnerabilities. While trust is equally foundational to the law, it has been neglected in both health care and laws affecting health care.[5]

This lack of trust is further justified by the recent reports of the significant number of medical errors that was reported by the Institute of Medicine. Its Project on the Quality of Healthcare in America was initiated in June 1998. The mission for the Project is to "develop a strategy that will result in a threshold improvement in quality over the next 10 years."[6] Data released reflect that deaths due to medical errors exceed the number of deaths attributable to the eighth leading cause of death, and increase health care costs by $8.5 billion–$14.5 billion. Any trust that existed previously between patients and the health care system, and in particular with nurses and physicians, has been significantly impacted.

---

2 Hall, M. A. *Law, Medicine, and Trust.* 9 Journal of Nursing Law 33 (2003).

3 Easterbrook, F. H. *Cyberspace and the Law of the Horse.* Univ. Chicago. Legal F. 207 (1996).

4 Wexler, D. B. and Winick, B. J. *Essays and Therapeutic Jurisprudence* (1991).

5 Hall, *supra* at 35.

6 Institute of Medicine, *supra* at 5.

Headlines in the newspaper only add to this mistrust: "Death from Overdose During Chemotherapy;" "Wrong Leg Amputated;" "Drug Mix-up Causes Death of 8-Year Old." National committees have issued similar reports: "There is increasing evidence of inappropriate medical care; overuse, underuse, and misuse of health care services are leading to adverse outcomes and unnecessary costs."[7]

So how do I remain optimistic? Because recent Gallup polls concluded that for the second year in a row, nurses are perceived as #1 by the public in honesty compared to other professions, such as pharmacists (#2), veterinarians (#3), and physicians (#4), and as #1 in ethical behavior which is the same rating as for the clergy.[8]

Nurses are health care's frontline professionals and constitute the largest health care profession in the United States at 2.7 million people. Research is demonstrating the high correlation between the number and kind of nurses delivering care and improved outcomes for patients. Nurses are the folks who *can* make health care safer for patients and who can improve the quality of life for patients, both of which will result in decreased health care costs. Being knowledgeable of therapeutic jurisprudence will best prepare you to meet your many challenges. The journey is ahead.

REFERENCES

Agency for Healthcare Research and Quality, *The AHRQ Web M&M* (a monthly web-based medical journal that highlights patient safety lessons taken from real life instances of medical errors), at http://www.webmm.ahrq.gov.

Call to the Nursing Profession and Nursing's Agenda for the Future Steering Committee, *Nurses Agenda for the Future,* American Nurses Association (2002).

Ellwood, P. M., *Crossing the Health Policy Chasm: Pathways to Healthy Outcomes,* at http://www.facct.org (2003).

---

7 Research and Policy Committee of the Committee for Economic Development, *A New Vision for Healthcare: A Leadership Role for Business.* Committee for Economic Development (2002).

8 Williams, S., *Split Decision: Nursing Profession Ranks Low in Desirability Despite Public's High Regard for Nurses.* Nurseweek (April 16, 2001); Joseph, L. and Lewis, A. *Who Has The Highest Ethics,* USA Today 1A (June 4, 2001).

CHAPTER 2

The Legal System and Principles

SECTION 2-1: SOURCES AND TYPES OF LAWS

A. Overview

The term "law" is derived from the Anglo-Saxon "lagu" which means that which is laid down or fixed. Laws regulate how society conducts itself. Because human interactions are complex and constantly changing, so are laws. Laws are enacted to address what threatens society at the moment.

In the United States, the supreme laws are the United Stated Constitution. The Constitution defines the operation of the Federal government and differentiates between powers and limitations of the Federal and State governments. The first ten Amendments to the Constitution are the Bill of Rights which protect certain individual rights, including free speech, religion, privacy, trial by jury, and due process of law. No other laws may infringe upon or conflict with constitutional provisions.

State laws cannot conflict with Federal laws; however, State laws may be stricter than Federal laws. State laws frequently address issues that have not been addressed in the Constitution or by the Federal government. Laws must be read and applied in conjunction with other laws, considering both State and Federal laws.

In addition to the United States Constitution, the other sources of laws are: (a) Statutes; (b) Regulations; (c) Common Law/Court Decisions; and (d) Attorney General Opinions.

All have equal force and affect, and establish precedents for future behavior.

B. Statutes

Statutes are rules that have been enacted by a legislative body and signed into law by either a State Governor or the President of the United States. Through statutes, regulatory agencies are established and given the power to act. Nurse Practice Acts are actually a series of State statutes that define and govern the practice of nursing within that State. These statutes establish the State regulatory board of nursing and give it authority to operate. Other statutes affecting nursing practice include child and elder neglect and abuse, statutes of limitations for filing lawsuits, civil detention procedures, guardianship, and consent for medical treatment.

Frequently courts must interpret statutes because they are not always written to mean what they say, or say what they mean. There are certain well established rules of statutory construction that courts rely upon. The initial focus is typically to ascertain the intent of the enacting legislative body so that the statute effectuates that purpose.[1] The words of the statute are examined since they are usually the most reliable indicator of legislative intent, and the words are given their ordinary and usual meaning.[2] The word "including" is typically interpreted as a term of enlargement rather than limitation.[3] When available, the legislative history or analysis by the legislative committee staff may be considered a determining legislative intent.[4]

C. Regulations

Regulations are rules enacted by regulatory agencies to further implement statutes and carry out their objectives. Because these agencies are usually composed of individuals with expertise in the particular area being regulated, they are deemed to be in the best position to more specifically regulate an activity. A State's regulatory agency for nurses, which is typically composed of nurses of various backgrounds, has the authority to establish curriculums for nursing education programs and certify them, establish criteria for obtaining licensure, and conduct investigations and hearings regarding potential violations of the Nurse Practice Act or regulations.

D. Common Law/Court Decisions

Common law is that which results from court decisions rather than from legislation. It is the result of courts recognizing and enforcing customs and social values. "As a product of the courts, the common law has developed case by case

---

1 *Hassan v. Mercy American River Hospital*, 74 P.3d 726, 3 Cal. Rptr.3d 623, 626 (Cal. 2003).

2 *Id.* at 626.

3 *Id.* at 627.

4 *Quelimane Company v. Stewart Title Guaranty Company*, 77 Cal. Rptr. 2d 709, 960 P.2d 513 (Cal. 1998).

in response to social needs; the common law has evolved gradually as society has changed and new rights have been recognized.[5]

Both State and Federal court decisions are important. There are two types of courts, trial courts and appellate courts, on the Federal and State levels. The trial court is where a lawsuit is initially filed. The purpose of the trial court is to decide issues of fact and to apply the law with either a judge or jury rendering a verdict.

If a party in the trial court action is not satisfied with the outcome, the party has the option of seeking an appeal from an appellate court. Appellate courts have different titles among States, but are generally referred to as "Court of Appeals" or "Superior Courts." The purpose of an appellate court is to decide difficult legal issues that may include interpreting statutes or regulations, reconciling conflicting laws, or determining whether Federal or State law should apply. Appellate courts consist only of judges who render opinions based upon legal arguments presented by attorneys for the parties. No factual witnesses or evidence are presented in appellate courts.

If an opinion rendered by an appellate court is not satisfactory to a party, that decision may be further appealed to the State Supreme Court.

The final court of action for both State and Federal courts is the United States Supreme Court. However, none of the appellate courts are compelled to review a trial court case. On a State level, its Supreme Court is the highest authority; its decisions are binding on all other courts in that State. Similarly, decisions rendered by the United States Supreme Court are binding on *all* trial and appellate courts on the State and Federal levels.

E. Attorney General Opinions

The Attorney General is the chief attorney for the State or Government. The Attorney General renders legal opinions usually where a statute or regulation or court decision is unclear and an individual wants to clarify the law. The amount of weight given to Attorney General opinions differs, but generally individuals may rely upon them. A State Attorney General is a resource for nurses who may question their authority to practice or perform certain functions under the authority of their State's Nurse Practice Act. Through a State legislator or nursing regulatory agency, a request can be made to the Attorney General for an opinion.

As Mae West once said, "It ain't no sin if you crack a few laws now and then, just so long as you don't break any." As you know, a very thin line frequently separates what is legal and illegal. That thin line is what precipitates lawsuits. To at least maximize that line, stay current with those laws affecting your specialty and practice location. Resources for this information include the American Nurses

---

5 *Lundman v. McKown*, 530 N.W.2d 807, 819 (Minn. App. 1995).

Association, State Nurses Associations, state nursing regulatory agency, publications of the specialty nursing organizations, and State Bar Associations.

SECTION 2-2: SCOPE OF LIABILITY

A. Historical Development of Nursing Liability

Throughout the 20th Century, not only has nursing changed significantly as a profession, but there have been equally significant changes in judicial standards for nurses. The increased professionalism has heightened the standards of care and enlarged the potential for liability. The earliest cases portray the nurse as a relatively menial member of the health care system who was perceived to primarily be a handmaiden to the physician and whose only task was to follow physician orders. Rarely were nurses named as defendants even when nursing care was the issue in a lawsuit; the target defendants were physicians and the employers of the nurses.

The earliest reported case of nursing negligence in which a nurse was personally named is *Isenstein v. Malcomson*[6] This is an action for personal injury sustained by a hospitalized patient due to negligence and carelessness of the nurse. The nurse was found to have "placed a hot water container against the limbs of the plaintiff at a time when she was unconscious, and allowed the container to remain on the limbs, with the hot water therein, for such a length of time that plaintiff (patient's) flesh was burned from her limbs to the bones."[7] The issue for the court was which standard of care was applicable to the nurse: malpractice or ordinary negligence. As the court noted, "malpractice" was commonly used to reflect improper treatment or neglect by a physician and had never been applied to a nurse. Thus, the court concluded: "nor is there anything in the text of this complaint which indicates that the gravamen of the action is other than the negligent conduct and reckless, careless, and incompetent performance of common duties of a person engaged in an employment for such specified duties, as distinguished from lack of or improper performance of work requiring purely professional skill."[8] Even in the 1950s courts were still ruling that "nurses in the discharge of their duties must obey and diligently execute the orders of the physician or surgeon in charge of the patient for nurses are not supposed to be experts in the techniques of diagnosis or the mechanics of treatment."[9]

---

6 236 N.Y.S. 641 (N.Y.App. 1929).

7 *Id.* at 641.

8 *Id.* at 643.

9 *McElroy v. Employers' Liability Assurance Corporation*, 163 F.Supp. 193, 198 (W.D.Ar. 1958).

In an analysis of nurses in litigation from 1990–1997, a research study identified seven patient-care-related categories of claims: (a) failure to ensure the safety of patients, visitors, and/or staff; (b) failure to exercise reasonable patient care; (c) inadequate communication; (d) criminal actions, emotional distress, and intentional torts; (e) failure to assess, analyze, and diagnose; (f) failure to take the appropriate action; and (g) failure to provide treatment.[10]

The majority of the litigation alleged a claim related to a nurses failure to take the appropriate action, which included the failure to initiate proper treatment as required by the patient's condition, failure to follow hospital policies, failure to use the correct equipment, failure to follow physician's orders, and failure to initiate appropriate monitoring.[11]

Nurses employed in obstetrics and gynecology had the highest percentage (15%) of the lawsuits. The area of perioperative nursing, which includes the preoperative unit, operating room, recovery room, and postoperative care unit, had the highest overall incidents of litigation (18.37%). Only a small percentage of cases (12.6%) occurred outside of hospitals, such as nursing homes, correctional facilities, home health care agencies, occupational centers, clinics or offices, and hospice agencies.[12]

B. Individual

Individuals are legally accountable for acts of negligence personally committed. *All* health care providers are accountable for their own actions: nurses, physicians, pharmacists, social workers, respiratory therapists, unlicensed assistive personnel, aides, technicians. Each is responsible for providing care within the appropriate standards of care for that provider. Health care providers are required to exercise independent judgments and utilize their knowledge within the scope of their profession or job when caring for patients.

Nurses are found liable with absolutely no liability placed upon a physician. Physicians and other health care providers are entitled to rely upon nurses to act competently. Where a nurse deviates from the acceptable standard of care and other health care providers act reasonably based upon that deviation, the sole accountability remains with the nurse.

In *Brennan v. Orlando Regional Healthcare Systems, Inc.*, an action was brought only against the defendant hospital on behalf of nursing malpractice.[13] The suit resulted from a premature birth caused by maternal staphylococcus

---

10 Smith-Pittman, M.H., *Nurses and Litigation: 1990–1997.* Journal of Nursing Law 7 (1998).

11 *Id.* at 15–16.

12 *Id.* at 12.

13 Case No. 95-2408 (Florida June 1999).

infection, resulting in a premature child who subsequently developed cerebral palsy. The mother was hospitalized for possible preterm labor and medications were administered IV to stop labor. After being hospitalized for 11 days, the IV site was red, swollen, and had a red streak extending 1.5 inches up the arm. The evidence was that the IV site was then changed for the first time. However, the nurse failed to notify the mother's treating physician. Three days later, the mother developed a sudden onset of fever, went into labor, and her daughter was born two hours thereafter. At trial, on behalf of the plaintiffs, the treating physician testified that had he been notified about the condition of the IV site, he would have started the mother on antibiotics which would have prevented the staph infection from developing and likely would have prevented the premature labor. The plaintiff's nursing expert testified that it was a deviation from the standards of nursing care for the nurses to have left the same IV in place for 11 days. The nurses further deviated from the standard of care by failing to notify the mother's physicians since there was clearly a risk for infection. The jury awarded the parents and their minor daughter, age 6 at the time of trial, $79,728 in past medical expenses, $6,061,996 in future rehabilitation care, $1,505,565 for future lost of wages, and $1,000,000 for future pain and suffering.

The plaintiff brought an action against the defendant OB/GYN as well as the hospital where her twins were delivered.[14] The allegation was that the defendant OB/GYN negligently caused injury to the umbilical court necessitating an emergency Caesarean Section, and that both the defendant OB/GYN and the nurses employed by the defendant hospital were negligent in leaving a sponge inside the plaintiff's abdominal cavity during the delivery. At trial, the defendant OB/GYN argued the nurses were responsible for providing an adequate sponge count and had performed three sponge counts after completion of the C-Section, reporting that the sponge counts were accurate. The plaintiff subsequently had surgery to remove the sponge but due to infection, a 3–4 foot section of bowel was removed, resulting in irritable bowel syndrome and panic attacks. The jury found that the defendant OB/GYN was *not* negligent and awarded $175,000 to the plaintiff against the defendant hospital only.

C. Third Party/Delegation to Others

The National Council of State Boards of Nursing, Inc. issued a paper in 1997 (which is current as of November 2003) outlining policies for acceptable delegation.[15] The need is obvious for competent, appropriately supervised, unlicensed health care workers to deliver affordable and quality health care. When

---

14 *Bartram v. Zafar, et al.*, Case No. 99-MP-1846 (Florida May 2001).

15 National Council of State Boards of Nursing, Inc., *Delegation: Concepts and Decision-Making Process*, at http://www.ncsbn.org/files/delegati.html.

a nurse delegates a task to another health care provider, whether the intent of that health care provider is to "assist" or "replace" the nurse depends upon the licensure status, competence, and purpose for delegation. Certain nursing tasks such as assessment, evaluation, and the exercise of nursing judgment cannot be delegated to an unlicensed health care worker. Any delegated task is expected to be performed consistent with established standards of practice, whether it is performed by a licensed or unlicensed health care provider.

In addition to the individual liability of a nurse, others may also be held accountable for the nurse's negligence. This liability is for the acts of a third party for whom an individual has management or administrative responsibilities. This *expands* liability; it does not relieve the individual nurse from personal liability.

This liability typically results when a nurse delegates duties to another nurse or unlicensed health care worker. Liability may be based on: (a) an inappropriate assignment or delegation of duties; or (b) inadequate supervision.

An *appropriate* assignment or delegation of duties means they were given to a provider who is qualified to carry out those tasks. The delegator has the right to rely upon the provider to carry out assigned tasks competently. This is true regardless of whether that provider is an R.N., L.P.N., L.V.N., nurse's aide, unlicensed assistive personnel, or the secretary. If the provider is not competent to carry out assigned tasks, then the delegator must provide *adequate* supervision for that provider. This includes having policies available for reference, periodically evaluating the provider's competency to perform assigned tasks, and providing direct supervision or oversight of the provider *if* there is a concern about competency. When an assignment is made to a competent provider and there is adequate supervision, the delegator will *not* be held liable for the acts of the provider.

D. Employer

Under a doctrine called vicarious liability or respondeat superior, employers are *automatically* liable for the acts of its employees. This is based upon public policy which encourages employers to hire competent employees and to provide them with the facilities, equipment, and staff needed to provide competent care to patients. If an employee performs negligently, the employer will vicariously or automatically be held accountable for that employee's negligence.

E. Corporate

The health care facility has its own responsibilities to patients for which it will be held accountable under corporate negligence. Many of the same responsibilities for which managers will be held accountable are also responsibilities of the facility. Because the facility acts through personnel, they will generally be the individuals against whom allegations of negligence are made and whose negligence will also constitute corporate negligence. Some examples of corporate responsibilities are: (a) hiring competent personnel; (b) providing education opportunities for the nursing staff, such as workshops and seminars; (c) having adequate library services accessible; (d) providing adequate and sufficient equipment and supplies as well as maintaining them; and (e) monitoring that personnel are carrying out their duties competently.

F. Independent Contractor

Independent contractors are individuals with special skills who are hired to perform specific jobs or for a specific period of employment. The distinction between an employee and an independent contractor is based on the amount of control the employer has over the individual. While an employer generally has the right of control over its employees and the employees are performing services as requested by the employer, independent contractors follow their own discretion in accomplishing a job. There is no right of control by the employer over an independent contractor and, therefore, generally no liability.

However, the employer has liability for the acts of an independent contractor if the employer is negligent in its duty of selecting a competent independent contractor and it is shown that there was or should have been prior knowledge of the incompetency of that individual. Because the independent contractor is being held out to the public by the employer, the duty is to provide a competent individual.

G. Captain-of-the-Ship

The doctrine of captain-of-the-ship as a basis for liability was first employed in the medical malpractice context in *McConnell v. Williams*.[16] In the Navy, the captain of the ship is in total command. Full responsibility for the care and efficiency of the ship and welfare for all hands is placed upon the captain. As a result, the captain must have supreme authority.

In applying this doctrine to medicine, complete responsibility is placed upon the surgeon in the operating suite for the acts of all those present and assisting during the operation. This includes acts of any residents or medical students, as well as those of circulating and scrub nurses. However, this doctrine has been abandoned in most States. Instead, any liability imposed upon a surgeon will be based upon one of the other legal relationships, such as the surgeon borrowing a servant or acting in a supervisory capacity.

---

16 65 A.2d 243 (Pa. 1949).

H. Student Nurses

The potential liability for student nurses is the same as that for licensed nurses. Student nurses must comply with the same standards of care as any licensed nurses practicing in that area. Student nurses are responsible for their own actions. Assignments for students must be made with the same consideration as assignments for other nurses; students must not be assigned tasks beyond their capabilities, and where necessary, adequate supervision must be provided.

The frequent issue is who has supervisory responsibilities for a student nurse: the student's clinical instructor or a nurse employee from the health care facility. If the instructor makes the student's assignments and supervise the student is the clinical area, then the instructor is accountable for assessing the student's capabilities and providing adequate supervision as needed by the student. If the nurse employee assumes the responsibility for supervising the student, the instructor must provide the nurse employee with information about the student and the student's capabilities, or the nurse employee must personally assess the competency of the student nurse to appropriately delegate duties and provide appropriate supervision.

Additionally, it must be made clear to patients that care is being provided by student nurses who *are not employees* of the health care facility. Otherwise, the apparent agency theory of liability may be raised against the facility (facility is holding student nurses out to patients as employees).

SECTION 2-3: CIVIL ACTIONS

A. Elements of Liability

Civil law is that area concerned with the rights and duties of private persons. For civil law violations, enforcement is sought by filing a lawsuit seeking money compensation or requesting the court to enforce a specific action to be performed. Civil law is divided into a variety of subareas: contract law; labor law; patent law; family law; and tort law.

A *tort* is a civil wrong committed by a person against another person or the property of another. Tort law is based on fault—something was done incorrectly or something was omitted from being done. Torts include negligence and intentional torts. Negligence denotes conduct lacking in due care, or carelessness. It is a deviation from the standard of care.

Intentional torts are differentiated from negligence by intent and these three elements:

    1. A volitional act;

2. The person intended to bring about the consequences or knew that they were likely to occur; and

3. The act must be a substantial factor in causing the injury or consequences.

For a plaintiff to prevail in a civil action requires proof of four elements. The burden of proving these is upon the plaintiff.

Duty

Duty is a legal relationship between a nurse and a patient requiring the nurse to provide a certain standard of care to that patient. The nurse-patient relationship must be established before the duty arises. Most frequently the duty arises when a nurse is assigned to a specific patient. However, it is also established if a nurse while working in the employment setting becomes aware of an unassigned patient needing assistance. That awareness establishes a duty whereby the nurse must either offer assistance or obtain the assistance needed by that patient. Duty arises in a third way: when a nurse observes another health care provider performing in a manner that may cause injury to a patient. This duty of affirmative action requires the nurse to not passively observe inferior care but to intervene on behalf of the patient. The appropriate amount of intervention required is dependent upon the facts of the situation as they relate to the patient's potential injury. But once a duty is created, the nurse becomes accountable to the patient.

When a 30 year old woman died of cardiac arrest following routine outpatient removal of a benign fibroid tumor in her uterus, at Beth Israel Hospital in Manhattan, New York, was found to have violated more than twelve medical standards, including permitting a sales representative to operate controls that regulated the amount of current being used in an electrical cauterizing tool during the procedure.[17] Prior to the procedure, the nurses in the operating room knew that the sales representative intended to operate the electrosurgery system which they knew was against Hospital Policy. The nurses were also being asked to use equipment for which they had no formal training. This is clearly the type of situation when nurses must refuse improper orders and notify management. "Absolutely, the nurses should know just from being a nurse that it's not right for a sales person to perform patient care. . . . they should have questioned the doctor's orders on the spot and then should have run right out and grabbed their OR supervisor. This certainly was out of the ordinary and they should have acted to protect the patient."[18] Even after the procedure began, the nurse noticed that the fluid was not properly draining and advised the physicians. The physicians said not to worry.

---

17 *Do You Have Right Policies for Sales Reps in OR?* Hospital Peer Review 24 (February 1999).
18 *Id.* at 25.

According to the report of the New York State Health Department, the excessive infusion of fluid was the cause of the patient's cardiac arrest and death.

On March 10, 1996, a patient was involved in a head-on collision and was taken to the Emergency Department of the defendant hospital for an evaluation by a trauma surgeon. The neurological evaluation was within normal limits; however, the patient had a fracture of the right femur and fractures of T12 and L1. On the following day, a nurse assessed the patient and determined that he could not move his right great toe and his left leg was somewhat weak. She reported it to the orthopedist. At noon on March 12, a pulmonary consultant saw the patient; he was informed by the patient's daughter about the patient's weakness to which he responded by telling the floor nurse to obtain a neurology consultation. Although the nurse quickly contacted a neurologist, he indicated that he didn't have privileges for trauma patients. The nurse then phoned the pulmonologist who told her to call the orthopedist. The nurse phoned the orthopedist but was unable to find him.

About midnight, the pulmonologist again came to see the patient. He telephoned the trauma surgeon with his concerns about the motor deficits and they agreed the patient should be immediately transferred to another hospital for definitive care. A neurosurgeon operated about 2:00 p.m. on March 13, stabilizing the fractures at T12 and L1. The patient sustained a moderate paralysis and has marginal bowel and bladder control. At trial, there was testimony that the nurse has an individual professional responsibility to a patient such that if a nurse recognizes that patient's condition is deteriorating, the nurse must take appropriate action when the physician is neglectful. Thus, it was the nurse's obligation to the patient, as early as Monday morning, to respond to the orthopedist's neglect of the new finding of a neurologic deficit by contacting a nursing supervisor, calling the Chief of Staff, etc."[19]

The jury deliberated 14 days before returning their verdict of $4.7 million, with 25% of the liability assigned to the Hospital for the negligence of its nurses.

A fundamental rule of American tort law is: *There is no duty to rescue.*[20] However, a duty can be voluntarily assumed. "One has, for example, no duty to drive one's neighbor to the airport. But if one nevertheless volunteers to undertake that good-neighborly task, and then drives negligently, causing the neighbor to be injured en route, one is held legally accountable."[21]

---

19 *A $4.7 million Verdict for Diagnostic Oversight,* 28 Professional Liability Newsletter 1 (October 1998).

20 Groninger, J. L. *No Duty to Rescue: Can Americans Really Leave a Victim Lying in the Street? What is Left of the American Rule, and Will It Survive Unbated?* 26 Pepperdine Law Review 353 (1999).

21 *Kotofsky v. Albert Enstein Medical Center,* 2000 WL 1618475 (E.D. Pa. 2000).

Negligence/Malpractice

The legal definition of the level of conduct for which a nurse is held accountable is the *standard of care*. It is that level of care that a reasonably prudent nurse would render under the same or similar circumstances. The standard of care is based on expected conduct by a similarly educated and experienced nurse with average intelligence, judgment, foresight, and skill. The majority of States recognize a minimum or national standard of care, i.e., a nurse practicing in Kansas can be expected to meet the same minimum standard of care as a nurse practicing in Washington, Texas, or Rhode Island.

The failure to meet the applicable standard of care results in negligence. When referring to the negligence of a professional, the term malpractice is normally used. Malpractice arises when the nurse's level of conduct falls below the appropriate standard of care for that nurse. Proof that a nurse committed malpractice usually requires the testimony of an expert nurse witness, an individual with the qualifications and expertise in the same area as that of the defendant nurse who can testify that the nurse's level of conduct fell below the standard of care required in that situation.

The standard of care for which a nurse is held accountable has evolved as the professionalism of nurses has increased. In the first reported case of nursing negligence, which involved physical injuries sustained by a hospitalized patient when the nurse placed a hot water container on the patient, causing burns, held that the standard of care for which the nurse is accountable is ordinary negligence. The standard was similar to that owed by lay persons.[22]

One of the earliest reported cases holding nurses to a malpractice standard is *Thompson v. United States*.[23] The court held that the nurses were expected to meet a standard of care consistent with the "exercise of the degree of skill ordinarily employed under similar circumstances by members of the nursing profession in good standing in the same community or locality."[24]

The other significant change in the standard of care has been from a local standard, or "locality rule," to a national standard of care. In *McMillan v. Durant*[25], the applicable standard of care for nurses was discussed by the Court. Joseph McMillan was born prematurely, suffered intercranial bleeding, and required the insertion of a shunt. He subsequently became ill and the pediatrician diagnosed him with an inflammation of the stomach and intestines. As a precaution for Joseph's dehydration, he was admitted to the hospital for intra-

---

22 *Isenstein v. Malcomson*, 236 NY.Supp. 641 (NY. App. 1929).

23 368 F.Supp. 466 (W.D.LA. 1973).

24 *Id.* at 468.

25 439 S.E.2d 829 (S.C. 1993).

venous hydration. The evening of his day of admission, Joseph was assessed several times by nurses while he was in his mother's arms in a semi-dark room and was apparently sleeping. The mother mentioned to the nurses that Joseph was not acting normally because he would open and close his mouth as he breathed. Shortly thereafter, Joseph stopped breathing and efforts to resuscitate him began immediately. The neurosurgeon decided to tap the shunt and, if excess pressure was found, to drain the excess fluid. Joseph's shunt was drained twice before the pressure was reduced to a safe level. Unfortunately Joseph sustained severe, permanent brain damage. At trial, the Hospital argued that the locality rule still applied as the appropriate standard of nursing care. However, the court noted that in 1981, a national standard of care for physicians and dentists in South Carolina was adopted, and the concerns for regional limits on training and lack of exposure to multi-regional practice for physicians was equally outdated for nurses. Several other States in the 1980s had extended the appropriate standard of care for physicians to nurses.[26] The court further noted that many other States had recognized nurses as health care professionals who should be subjected to the same standards as other health care providers. The jury found that the nurses failed to recognize the significance of Joseph's abnormal breathing and made no attempt to contact a physician. The jury returned a verdict in favor of plaintiffs for $734,100.

One State that continues to use a locality rule is Louisiana.[27] Louisiana defines the standard of care required of health care providers, excluding hospitals, nursing homes, offices, and clinics, in rendering professional services or health care to a patient to be that degree of skill ordinarily employed, under similar circumstances, by other members in the profession in the same community or locality, and to use reasonable care and diligence, along with best judgment, in the application of skills. The difference between the standard of care for nurses from hospitals was addressed by the court in *Thomas v. Southwest Louisiana Hospital Association.*[28] This is an action where the patient brought suit against the hospital due to a fall she suffered from the hospital bed.

Under certain State laws, the standard for liability may be *gross* negligence, as it was in *Stewart v. Richland Memorial Hospital.*[29] The Tort Claims Act in South Carolina grants sovereign immunity to the state, its agencies, political subdivisions, and other governmental entities.[30] "Sovereign immunity" is a com-

---

26 *Durflinger v. Artiles*, 673 P.2d 86 (Kansas 1983); *Belmon v. St. Frances Cabrini Hospital*, 427 S.2d 541 (LA.App. 3 1983).

27 LaR.S. 40:1299.41(A)(7).

28 833 So.2d 548 (La.App. 3rd Cir. 2002).

29 567 S.E.2d 510 (S.C.App. 2002).

30 S.C. Code Ann.§ 15-78-40.

mon immunity available to governmental entities. In South Carolina, it is not available when the responsibility or duty is exercised in a grossly negligent manner.[31] In this case, the allegation was that the nurse breached the standard of care by removing the patient's restraints and failing to monitor him following surgery, which caused him injury. The Hospital was held not liable because the plaintiff failed to prove that the nurse acted in a grossly negligent manner.

Standards of care are flexible and constantly changing. They reflect advancements in medicine and nursing that affect patient care. Therefore, nurses are expected to keep current with the standards affecting their individual practices. Maintaining currency and competency requires continually updating knowledge, skills, and responsibilities. Nurses are held accountable for the standards of care that exist at the time they are delivering that care, not what they may have learned in nursing school one year, five years, or twenty years previously.

Written standards of care are used as evidence in malpractice trials by the plaintiff to prove in black and white that a nurse performed negligently. They become trial exhibits that are shown to the jury to demonstrate the conduct for which the nurse is to be held accountable.

Sources of standards are external and internal. State and Federal laws, and Standards of the Joint Commission on Accreditation of Healthcare Organizations, American Osteopathic Association, and National Committee for Quality Assurance are examples of external standards. Professional journals are also sources of external standards of care.

Nurses are responsible for developing guidelines and standards for specialized practices. Professional standards evolve from the scope of nursing practice and provide a framework for the development of competency statements. The ANA and most of the specialty nursing associations have written standards of care which establish that minimum level of conduct for which a nurse will be held accountable. A nurse working in a given area is required to meet the minimum standards of care for that specialty practice, even if that is not the nurse's normal assignment, or the nurse is not certified by or a member of the applicable nursing association.

Internal standards are those established by and for individual health care facilities. Frequently these more specifically define and individualize external standards of care as they pertain to that facility, that patient population, that nursing staff. Examples of internal standards of care include job descriptions, policies, and protocols. If internal standards establish higher standards of care than the minimum standards, they are the standards for which the facility's nurses are accountable. Therefore, utilize external standards of care when developing internal standards, both to ensure that minimum standards of care

---

31 S.C. Code Ann. § 115-78-60 (25).

are established for the facility, as well as to ensure that unrealistic higher standards of care are not established inadvertently. Facility standards of care must reflect *current* nursing practice, not future or wishful goals.

Causation of Injury

As a result of the nurse's negligence, the patient must sustain an injury. This is also referred to as proximate cause. Merely because a nurse performs negligently does not mean that the nurse will be held liable for any injury the patient sustains; rather, the injury must be caused by or the direct result of the nurse's negligence. Proof of causation requires the testimony of an expert witness, usually a physician, who can testify that but for the nurse's negligence the injury would not have occurred. This is the most difficult element for a plaintiff to prove because it may not be obvious, and there may be many viable explanations for the ultimate injury, only one of which may be the nurse's negligence. The standard of proving causation for a malpractice case is that the judge or jury must find that it is more probable that the causation of the injury was attributable to the nurse's negligence than it being attributable to any other cause.

Damages

Plaintiffs are entitled to seek compensation for any injuries sustained. Compensable damages are awarded for physical, financial, and emotional injuries. In an action for malpractice, the plaintiff must sustain damages as a result of the injury; otherwise, there is nothing for which to compensate the plaintiff. Damages may include both past losses and future losses.

If damages are awarded that a court determines "shock the conscience" the court may determine that remittitur is warranted. This was the position of the court in *Advocat, Inc. v. Sauer.*[32] Remittitur is a procedural process by which a jury verdict is diminished by subtraction, or the court may order a complete new trial or a trial limited to the issue of damages. In this action, Margaretha Sauer, 93 years old, was a resident at Ridge Mountain Nursing and Rehabilitation Center. On July 6, 1998, she was scheduled for the insertion of a gastrointestinal feeding tube into her stomach but the surgery was delayed. On July 18, a nursing note reflected that Ms. Sauer's vital signs began to decline, and on July 19, at 3:30 a.m., her vital signs were still declining and she wasn't acting right. At 5:00 a.m. that morning, a nurse reported the assessment of Ms. Sauer to her treating physician who ordered that she be taken immediately to an emergency room. By the time she arrived at the hospital, she was semi-comatose, and died about 16 hours later. At the time of her death, Ms. Sauer had lost 15 lbs in the

---

32 111 S.W.3d 346 (Ark. 2003).

last month and was in obvious need of a feeding tube. The cause of her death was severe malnutrition and dehydration.

Evidence at trial was that frequently Ms. Sauer's foodtray was in her room untouched because there was no staff member available to feed her. There was also testimony about numerous deficiencies, some of which were introduced through surveys from the State Office of Long-Term Care. The surveys were replete with statements about the lack of staffing to feed, bathe, and clean residents. Ms. Sauer's family testified how they frequently found their mother: with dried feces under her fingernails from scratching herself while lying in her own excrement; found at 3:00 p.m. still in her gown, wet with urine, disturbed and upset; not enough hot water to shower; suffering from poor oral hygiene with caked food and debris in her mouth. A former staff member also testified that at one time Ms. Sauer had a pressure sore the size of a softball, which was open, and had pressure sores on her back, lower buttock, and arms. Testimony of a former Regional Vice President for the Corporation that owned Ridge Mountain was that in 1996 the Corporate philosophy changed to stress profits over care. Finally, there was testimony that Ridge Mountain tried to cover up short staffing by false charting to show more staff than were actually present.

The jury returned a verdict for the plaintiffs on all counts submitted. It awarded compensatory damages of $5 million for ordinary negligence, $10 million for medical malpractice, $25,000 for breach of contract, and $100,000 for each of the surviving beneficiaries for wrongful death. Punitive damages in the amount of $21 million were awarded against each of the three defendants for a total punitive damage award of $63 million. The combined judgments totaled $78,425,000.00. This was the largest personal injury verdict ever awarded in Arkansas. The focus of review for the court was whether the damages awarded were excessive such as to shock the conscience of the court or demonstrate passion or prejudice by the jury. The court concluded that the jury verdicts were not based on passion or prejudice, but on the significant testimony that Ms. Sauer was not properly cared for, that Ridge Mountain was short staffed, and that Ridge Mountain tried to cover this up by false charting and by bringing in additional "employees" on State inspection days. Thus, there was sufficient evidence that Ridge Mountain and its owners knew it had staffing problems and yet allowed negligent care of Ms. Sauer to avoid incurring additional costs. "Compensation for pain and suffering must be left to the sound discretion of the jury and the conclusion reached by it should not be disturbed unless the award is clearly excessive."[33] The court concluded that while they were not the result of passion or prejudice, the compensatory damages awarded shocked the

---

33 *Id.* at 354.

conscience of the court. Remittitur was granted and the total damage award for negligence and malpractice was reduced from $15 million to $5 million.

The court then examined whether the punitive damages awarded were also excessive. When considering the issue of remittitur of punitive damages, "we consider the extent and enormity of the wrong, the intent of the party committing the wrong, all of the circumstances, and the financial and social condition and standing of the erring party."[34] The criteria used to determine whether an award of punitive damages is grossly excessive and violates due process are: (a) the degree of reprehensibility of the defendants' conduct; (b) the disparity between the harm or potential harm suffered by the plaintiff and the punitive damages award; (c) the difference between this remedy and the civil penalties authorized by statute or imposed in comparable cases. In assessing reprehensibility, factors to be considered include whether the harm caused was physical as opposed to economic; whether the tortuous conduct events an indifference to or a reckless disregard of the health or safety of others; whether the conduct was an isolated incident or involved repeated actions; and whether the harm was a result of intentional malice, trickery, deceit or mere accident. The court concluded that the harm inflicted upon Ms. Sauer certainly was physical, it was the budgetary constraints that contributed to the short staffing and inadequate supplies, the defendants were aware of the understaffing and yet it continued even after complaints from staff members, patients, family members, and the Office of Long-Term Care, and there were deliberate false entries on patient charts and efforts to conceal this evidence. The court concluded the reprehensibility of the defendants' conduct in this case was extremely high. However, because the three-named defendants were a parent company and two subsidiary companies, the court concluded that it was unreasonable to award the same amount of punitive damages against each defendant who in essence were one of the same; therefore, the court granted the remittitur and reduced the amount of punitive damages by two-thirds to $21 million.

B. Res Ipsa Loquitor

Res ipsa loquitor is not a doctrine of substantive law or a theory of recovery; rather, it is a rule allowing an inference regarding negligence to be made based on circumstantial evidence. "If common knowledge and experience leads one, in reviewing a situation, to realize that the situation would not normally occur without negligence, res ipsa loquitor exists to create the inference of negligence."[35] This doctrine is frequently applied where a sponge or medical device

---

34 *Id.* at 258.

35 Wampler, A. T. *Fly in the Buttermilk: Tennessee's Desire to Dispense with Lay Person Common Sense in the Medical Malpractice Locality Rule.* 69 Tennessee Law Review 385 (Winter 2002).

is left inside a patient during surgery or when an eye is cut during an appendectomy. There must still be evidence of all of the necessary elements for liability and the evidence must meet the burden of proof that more likely then not the injury was a result of the breach of the defendants' duty. This inference is one for the jury to determine.

In *Ybarra v. Spanguard,* the court discussed the purpose of this doctrine and how it benefits patients.[36] "Without the aid of the doctrine, a patient who receives permanent injuries of a serious character, obviously the result of someone's negligence, would be entirely unable to recover unless the doctors and nurses in attendance voluntarily chose to disclose the identity of the negligent person and the facts establishing liability."[37] The California Supreme Court identified the three conditions required to apply the doctrine of res ipsa loquitor: (a) the accident must be of a kind which ordinarily does not occur in the absent of someone's negligence; (b) it must be caused by an agency or instrumentality within the exclusive control of the defendants; and (c) it must have not been due to any voluntary action or contribution on the part of the plaintiff.

Expert witnesses are not required to establish standards of care where the doctrine of res ipsa loquitor applies. "In res ipsa cases, plaintiff need only prove his injury, and need not prove a standard of care or a specific act or omission."[38] Res ipsa loquitor is sometimes referred to as the doctrine of common knowledge because the facts are such that the common knowledge and experience possessed by lay persons enable the jury to conclude, without expert testimony, that a duty of care has been breached.

C. Intentional Torts

The other type of torts for which nurses may be held liable are intentional torts. These are acts that are performed by a nurse with the *intent* to bring about the result, or acts a nurse *should know* are likely to produce such a result. The result has to be *foreseeable*.

Assault and Battery

Assault is the unjustifiable *attempt* to touch another person or the threat of doing so, while battery is the actual *carrying out* of the threatened physical contact. To prove assault or battery requires evidence of the absence of consent. The distinction between battery and lack of informed consent, and whether the action

---

36   154 P.2d 687 (Cal. 1944).

37   *Id.* at 689.

38   *Estate of Chin v. St. Barnabas Medical Center,* 711 A.2d 352 (N.J. Super. 1998).

is an intentional tort or negligence, is based on if there has been any attempt to obtain the patient's consent. Where there is *no consent* given, the action will be one of *battery*. *Lack of informed consent* arises where there is not consent for the specific procedure performed, consent was obtained without full disclosure of the information necessary for the patient to make an informed decision, or the patient did not consent to the procedure being performed by that individual, and is negligence.

Defamation

Defamation occurs when a nurse discusses a patient in terms that diminish or harm the patient's reputation or business. *Libel* is written defamation while *slander* is oral defamation. To prove defamation requires three elements:

1. Actual damage to a reputation or business;
2. Must be communicated to a third person; and
3. Must be false.

However, many States also statutorily define certain statements as slanderous that do not require specific financial injury to allow compensation to the plaintiff. Such statements generally pertain to:

1. A contagious or venereal disease;
2. A crime involving moral turpitude; or
3. Fornication or adultery.

Invasion of Privacy

It is a constitutional right of every patient to be left alone. Violation of this right will result in a claim for invasion of privacy. This right of privacy protects a patient from:

1. Intrusion on the patient's physical or mental solitude and seclusion;
2. Public disclosure of private facts;
3. Publicity placing the patient in a false light in the public eye; and
4. Appropriation of the patient's name or likeness for the benefit or advantage of another.

In an action for invasion of privacy, a patient is entitled to recover merely because this right of privacy has been invaded, even *without showing* that any specific damages were sustained. The violation of the patient's right is damage in and of itself.

23

False Imprisonment

False imprisonment is an infringement of a patient's freedom of movement without justification. This typically involves psychiatric patients or the use of restraints. The issue to prove false imprisonment: the infringement was *not* justified. The patient's health information must reflect the facts relied upon to make the decision to restrict the patient's movement. False imprisonment is also an action that may be alleged as either a *negligent* action for confinement or the improper use of restraints, or an *intentional tort* if it is an unlawful restraint or if it is foreseeable that the injury would occur to the patient because of the restraints.

SECTION 2-4: DEFENSES

Defenses are legal justifications to escape liability. They may be legal or factual, or a combination of both. "Ignorance" is *not* a viable defense in a lawsuit! While the old adage "ignorance is bliss" may benefit some aspects of your life, it does *not* benefit you legally. Blissful ignorance results in legal liability!

A. Contributory or Comparative Negligence

Contributory or comparative negligence is a defense whereby the acts of the patient are examined to determine if they caused or contributed to the injury sustained by the patient. Contributory negligence traditionally barred a plaintiff's right to recovery if it could be shown that the plaintiff contributed to the ultimate injury. Most States now recognize the defense of comparative negligence which allows the jury to apportion liability among the parties, but does not completely bar the plaintiff from recovery. If liability is apportioned, the plaintiff's damages are then diminished by any percentage of fault assessed against the plaintiff. Other States have combined these defenses—if a plaintiff is assessed more than 50% of fault, that prevents the plaintiff from recovering damages.

A jury had no hesitancy in finding that the patient contributed to her development of thrombophlebitis in *Nordt v. Wenck.*[39] In November 1988, Mary Wenck broke her right leg. She was treated by Dr. Nordt for a major fracture of the two bones between the knee and ankle. Dr. Nordt placed a cast on her leg that reached from her foot to her groin. Dr. Nordt was concerned that Ms. Wenck could be at risk for developing either thrombophlebitis or compartment syndrome. However, he did not treat her with anticoagulant drugs because he feared those might increase the bleeding at the fracture site, thereby increasing Ms. Wenck's risk of developing compartment syndrome. As an alternative, he prescribed elevation of her legs and physical therapy.

---

39 653 So.2d 450 (Fla. App. 1995).

On December 1, 1988, Ms. Wenck was released from the hospital and ordered to continue physical therapy. Frequently she refused the therapy, claiming that it was uncomfortable, and complained of pain and swelling. Dr. Nordt examined Ms. Wenck twice after her release but failed to see any symptoms or diagnose any problem.

On January 1, 1989, Ms. Wenck called Dr. Nordt because she was feeling extremely ill and had swelling in both legs. Ms. Wenck was diagnosed as having thrombophlebitis with clots in both legs up both sides of her body to just below her kidneys. A Greenfield filter to prevent blood clots from going to her lungs was inserted and she was placed on anticoagulant therapy.

Ms. Wenck sued Dr. Nordt for malpractice for failing to prevent the onset of thrombophlebitis, failing to diagnose the condition as it progressed, and failing to treat the condition after symptoms manifested.

At trial, Dr. Nordt presented testimony that Ms. Wenck was negligent for failing to comply with his treatment and discharge instructions, and that such noncompliance contributed to her injury. On cross-examination, Ms. Wenck admitted that during her recovery, contrary to Dr. Nordt's advice, she had not performed her physical therapy, she had not maintained her legs in an elevated position above her heart, and she had not quit smoking. She further testified that during the last three or four days preceding the thrombophlebitis, she had "just laid there" and had "no activity."

Two expert witnesses testified that, within a reasonable medical probability, Ms. Wenck did not have deep venous thrombosis when she was discharged from the hospital. In their opinion, Ms. Wenck's inactivity triggered or enhanced the thrombophlebitis, and had she followed Dr. Nordt's instructions, remained active, and performed the prescribed physical therapy, her thrombophlebitis would have been avoided.

B. Statute of Limitations

The statute of limitations is the period of time established by State law in which injured patients must file lawsuits.

Depending on the State law, the statute begins running either the *date* of the incident causing the harm or when the patient *knows* or *should have known* that an injury may have been caused by negligence. Some States limit actions is and to a certain date beyond the date of the incident.[40] This limits the time a lawsuit can be initiated to allow a defendant the best opportunity to defend itself so that

---

40 Kan.Stat.Ann. § 60-513(c) (maximum time to bring a lawsuit is 4 years from the date of the incident).

pertinent people are still available and facts can be recollected. The time limit is typically extended if the patient is a minor at the time of the incident.[41]

Other legal acts have different statutes of limitations, such as product liability, wrongful death, and foreign objects left inside a patient. However, when the time period expires, the patient is then legally barred from filing a lawsuit (unless there has been fraud or misrepresentation to the patient which may extend the time period).

The applicable statute of limitations caused Nurse Malcomson to be subject to a lawsuit.[42] The issue of what standard of care the nurse was required to meet determined which statute of limitations was applicable. Actions for malpractice had to be filed within 2 years, while actions for negligence had to be filed within 3 years. As a result of the court's holding that the malpractice standard of care didn't apply to nurses, the patient was entitled to pursue the claim. (The conduct of the nurse must only meet a "negligent" standard of care, i.e., reckless, careless, incompetent performance or common duties as distinguished from lack of improper performance of work requiring professional skills).[43]

C. Sovereign Immunity

Sovereign immunity is a common law doctrine providing immunity to governmental agencies to avoid liability. It protects County, Municipal, City, and State health care agencies and institutions from being sued for malpractice. It is based upon the old English notion that the king can do no wrong; because of the king's sovereignty, he cannot be sued. In many States, sovereign immunity has been abolished or limited. It doesn't always restrict lawsuits against the individual employees of governmental agencies and facilities.

In South Carolina, sovereign immunity is still applicable to governmental entities, subject to certain limitations and exemptions.[44] The patient brought an action against the hospital alleging the nurse breached the standard of care by removing his restraints and failing to monitor him.[45] The patient subsequently fell from his bed and fractured his left hip. One of the exceptions for the immunity is gross negligence; therefore, the patient had to prove what was the standard of care, and that the nurse was grossly negligent in meeting that standard of care. Only then, would the immunity for the hospital be waived.

---

41 In Missouri, the statute of limitations for an injury to a minor extends until the minor is age 20. Mo.R.S. § 516.105(3).

42 *Isenstein v. Malcomson*, 236 N.Y.S. 641 (N.Y.App. 1929).

43 *Id.* at 643.

44 S.C. Code Ann. § 15-78-40.

45 *Stewart v. Richland Hospital*, 567 S.E.2d 510 (SC.App. 2002).

D. Good Samaritan Law

The term "Good Samaritan" derives from a New Testament parable in which a Samaritan was the only passer-by to aid a man who had been left dead by thieves.[46]

Because there is no legal duty to rescue, to encourage health care providers to stop and render assistance at the scene of an accident or disaster, since 1959 all States and the District of Columbia have enacted Good Samaritan Laws, with West Virginia being the most recent.[47] Some States extend protection only to licensed health care providers while others protect any citizen who stops to render assistance. Most States require that the assistance to be rendered gratuitously to be afforded the protection under the Good Samaritan Law.

Although the laws vary greatly among the States, generally they prevent liability for rendering *negligent* care but do not protect gross misconduct or willful or wanton conduct that causes harm to an individual. Thus, health care providers can be sued for rendering assistance and the jury must determine whether there was negligence or gross misconduct.

Courts are now addressing questions as to when does the Good Samaritan Law apply; what constitutes "the scene of an emergency." This was the question addressed by the Court in *Glorioso v. Police Department of Town of Burlington.*[48] The Hospital and Police Department were sued in connection with their responses to an emergency call for medical attention, with the allegation being gross negligence and reckless, wanton, or willful misconduct. The Hospital asserted that it was immune from liability under the Good Samaritan Law. The plaintiff's claims were that the Hospital's personnel were grossly negligent by: knowingly failing to respond to the 911 call in a timely manner; knowingly failed to perform CPR immediately; discharging or refusing assistance from others on the scene; fail to perform advanced life support and CPR simultaneously; fail to know where the ambulance was; failing to timely contact the hospital for advice; failing to properly intubate the patient; and failing to follow proper protocols. In Connecticut, the Good Samaritan Law provides that certain providers of emergency health care "shall not be liable to . . . (a) person assisted for civil damages for any personal injuries which result from acts or omissions by such person in rending the emergency care, which may constitute ordinary negligence." The law further states that "the immunity provided in the subsection does not apply to acts or omissions constituting gross, willful or wanton negligence."[49] The court agreed

---

46 Luke 10:30–37.

47 Mayo, T.A., *Health Care Law.* 55 SMU Law Review 1113 (Summer 2002); *Velazquez v. Jiminez, M.D.,* 798 A.2d 51, 247–251 (N.J. 2002).

48 826 S.2d 271 (Conn. Super. 2003).

49 C.G.S.A. § 52-557(b).

that the Good Samaritan Law did not abolish liability for gross negligence and gross negligence could be determined if the defendant engaged in a blatant degree of negligence that was "wanton, willful, reckless, and intentional misconduct." "There is a real difference between negligently failing to respond to a call for emergency aid and intentionally failing to do so. . . . The plaintiff had alleged a conscious decision by the Hospital not to respond to the call for emergency services, not to allow others at the scene to assist, not to administer CPR for an extended period of time, and other intentional withholding of needed care. These facts sufficiently state a claim of reckless, wanton, or willful misconduct."[50]

The New Jersey Supreme Court addressed whether the Good Samaritan Law can be invoked to immunize a physician who assists a patient at the hospital during a medical emergency.[51] Ms. Velazquez was at the Medical Center for the delivery of her baby. Her attending physician was Dr. Jiminez. When complications occurred during the delivery, Dr. Jiminez requested assistance from Dr. Ranzini. Dr. Ranzini subsequently delivered the baby by emergency Caesarean Section. The baby was born severely brain damaged, and died of pneumonia before reaching his third birthday. Dr. Ranzini argued that she was immunized from liability under the Good Samaritan Law; that the law didn't stop at the door at the hospital. As the court noted, "no two States are alike" in the provisions of the Good Samaritan Laws, including varying degrees of immunity to different classes of rescuers under a multitude of settings. Some laws unequivocally exclude from statutory immunity emergency care rendered to patients within a hospital or other health care facility. However, in seven states, emergency care provided in a hospital setting is immunized under Good Samaritan Laws.[52] After analyzing a significant number of the different Good Samaritan Laws, the Court concluded: "It would be fair to say that there is no universal interpretation of general statutory language among our sister jurisdictions, no road map to follow."[53] Know the extent of coverage that the Good Samaritan Law in your State provides.

SECTION 2-5: CRIMINAL ACTIONS

A recent trend has emerged significantly increasing criminal actions brought against nurses and other health care providers. In particular, they are being charged with crimes as a result of medical decisions and errors, such as over or under prescribing pain medication, treatment of wounds, and transfer decisions.

50 *Id.* at 276.
51 *Velazquez v. Jiminez, M.D.*, 798 A.2d, 51 (N.j. 2002).
52 *Id.* at 251.
53 *Id.* at 256.

Nurses are now often in the headlines for criminal acts. In June 2002, Regina Waites, a private duty home health nurse, was given a three year prison sentence for submitting timesheets for work not performed, resulting in a guilty plea to one count of Medicaid Health Plan Fraud.[54] Nurse Waites must also repay $126,706.00 to the Maryland Department of Health and Mental Hygiene.

A home health aid is accused of swindling a 91 year old client who suffered from dementia. She is charged with second degree grand larceny, second degree forgery, and second degree criminal possession of a forged instrument for allegedly writing 105 checks worth $166,673.00 which she convinced her client to sign. If convicted, she could face 15 years in prison.[55]

There has also been an aggressive approach to identifying Medicare and Medicaid fraud to recapture money paid illegally, which is a significant source of income for our Medicare and Medicaid Programs.

A. Healthcare Fraud

In 1996, the Healthcare Fraud and Abuse Control Program was established to combat fraud and abuse in health care. The money recovered from health care investigations, including criminal finds, forfeitures, civil settlements and judgments, and administrative penalties are deposited in the Medicare Trust Fund which is used to financial anti-fraud activities and to administer Federal health care programs. In 2001, the Federal government collected a record high of more than $1.3 billion in connection with health care fraud.[56] The detection and elimination of health care fraud and abuse is a top priority of both Federal and State governments. As the result of a successful collaboration between Federal and State governments and agencies, a record number of 3,756 individuals and entities were excluded from participating in the Medicare and Medicaid Programs as a result of convictions for crimes relating to Medicare or Medicaid, patient abuse or neglect, or as a result of licensure revocations.[57] The highlights for 2001 include:

- National Healthcare Corporation entered a $27 million civil settlement to resolve allegations of submitting inflated Medicare cost reports that overstated the number of hours that the nursing staff spent caring for Medicare patients and for billing or performing therapy that was not performed.

---

54 *Private Duty Nurse Who Billed Four Different Employers for Same Hours Gets One Year in Prison*, Home Health Line (June 28, 2002); at http://www.myhomehealth.com.

55 *Id.*

56 The Department of Health and Human Services and the Department of Justice, *Health Care Fraud and Abuse Control Program Annual Report for FY 2001* (April 2002), at http://oig.hhs.gov/publication/docs/hcfac/HCFAC%20Annual%20Report%20FY%202001.

57 *Id.*

- Manner Care, Inc. and affiliates settled a civil false claims act arising from alleged inadequate care at a skilled nursing facility, including substandard quality of patient care, inadequate care of pressure ulcers, insufficient staffing, training and supervision, and missing or incomplete assessments of the functional capacity and needs of residents. The company paid $90,000 and is required to retain an independent consultant to closely monitor future quality of care at the facility.

- A study of Medicare payments for mental health services reveal that 39% of psychiatric services in nursing homes were medically unnecessary, had no mental health documentation, or were questionable which may have cost $30 million. CMS has agreed to develop guidelines in these areas.

- Seven hospitals agreed to pay almost $5.5 million to settle claims that they unlawfully charged the Medicare and TRICARE programs for surgical procedures using experimental cardiac devices.

B. False Claims Act/Federal Criminal Actions

False certification lawsuits are brought under the False Claims Act.[58] A critical issue with Federal health programs is that the government is to pay only for services that are *medically reasonable and necessary*. Many of the cases involve certification arguments. When there is a failure of care such as the level or quality of care drops where it is not reasonable care anymore, resulting in the patient receiving inappropriate care, submitting payment for that care violates the certification that "reasonable and necessary services have been provided." This is the basis for making failure of care actionable under the False Claims Act.

In *United States v. NHC Healthcare*, a nursing home was sued for making false claims to Medicaid and Medicare programs for patient services and benefits that were either inadequate or not rendered at all.[59] The evidence was that the nursing home had such low staffing levels that it wasn't meeting the level of quality care that the government was paying for. While the court addressed the debate about the propriety of using the False Claims Act to evaluate quality of care, it held that quality of care can involve questions of whether necessary services were being performed and whether patients were actually being endangered.

For any criminal offenses related to the delivery of an item or service under a Federal health care program, the law *mandates* exclusion of health care providers from participation in Federal health care programs for a period of at

---

58   31 U.S.C. § 3728 et. seq.

59   115 F.Supp.2d 1149 (W.D.Mo. 2000).

least five years.[60] The effective result of this mandatory exclusion is that nurses are virtually unemployable for the period of exclusion since any health care services rendered by such nurses cannot be billed to a Federal health care program. Many private health care insurance companies have a similar exclusion. The Departmental Appeals Board of the Department of Health and Human Services is the administrative agency that handles questions related to the applicability of the mandatory exclusion for crimes related to a Federal health care program.

CAN Woodrum appealed her mandatory exclusion from participation in Federal health care programs for five years.[61] Woodrum was a licensed nursing assistant who provided home health nursing care services. She was found guilty in the District Court of Vermont of petit larceny for stealing $30.50 from the home of a daughter of a Medicare beneficiary. She was sentenced to probation, fined, and ordered to pay restitution in the amount of $30.50. CAN Woodrum argued that since her conviction was for a misdemeanor, the mandatory exclusion provision was not applicable. She further argued that she did not steal from Medicare or any other Federal health care program, nor did she steal from a Medicare beneficiary. She stole from the beneficiary's daughter. She therefore raised the question whether the criminal offense was related to the delivery of a health care item or service under a Federal health care program. The Administrative Law Judge concluded: "Theft of personal belongings violates professional standards of care expected of a nurse's aid. The expectation that petitioner would not steal personal property from patients under her care was an integral element of the services she provided to her patients."[62] Thus, the Administrative Law Judge upheld the mandatory exclusion for five years.

Michelle Thomas, a licensed practical nurse, pled guilty to one count of gross neglect of a patient for abusing a patient in a nursing home.[63] The Ohio State Court sentenced Nurse Thomas to 90 days in jail, which was suspended, three years probation, and a fine of $500. At the hearing, Nurse Thomas argued the propriety of her criminal conviction and asserted that she was not guilty of the act alleged. The Departmental Appeals Board has repeatedly held such arguments to be ineffectual in the context of an exclusion appeal since neither the Inspector General or the Administrative Law Judge are permitted to question the fact of conviction. Although the conviction was a misdemeanor offense, it did not preclude the imposition of the exclusion. The Administrative Law Judge held that the five year exclusion was mandatory because Nurse Thomas was

---

60 42 U.S.C. § 1320(a)-7.

61 *In the case of: Dorothy A. Woodrum v. The Inspector General*, DAB No. CR956 (2002).

62 *Id.*

63 *In the case of: Thomas v. The Inspector General*, DAB No. CR569 (January 29, 1999).

convicted of a criminal offense relating to the abuse or neglect of a patient in connection with the delivery of a health care item or service.

Nurse Michelle Burnette argued that the exclusive of five years from participating in federal health care programs was substantially greater than the two years of probation imposed upon her nursing license by the South Dakota Board of Nursing.[64] Nurse Burnette, a registered nurse, was involved in two incidents at the nursing home where she worked. One incident resulted in a felony offense of abuse of a disabled adult, and the other incident involved a misdemeanor offense of simple assault. Neither incident resulted in serious bodily injury to the residents. However, Nurse Burnette entered into a plea of no contest to the charge of simple assault and was sentenced to serve 15 days in jail. Nurse Burnette questioned whether the plea of no contest constituted a conviction as defined in the mandatory exclusion law. The Administrative Law Judge noted that to justify the exclusion, there must be evidence that: (1) the individual charged has been convicted of a criminal offense; (2) the conviction is related to the neglect abuse of a patient; and (3) the patient neglect abuse to which an excluded individual's conviction is related occurred in connection with the delivery of a health care item or service. The Administrative Law Judge concluded that a conviction of an offense based on charges of abusive conduct is sufficient, especially where the allegation was that she intentionally caused bodily injury to another in an incident. Furthermore, the term "abuse" is intended to include situations where a party willfully mistreats another person, which certainly includes physical assault. As the Administrative Law Judge noted, "It is well settled that the primary purpose of an exclusion is remedial rather than punitive. The purpose of a mandatory exclusion is to protect the integrity of the Medicare and Medicaid Programs, Program beneficiaries and recipients, and the public from persons who have been shown to be guilty of Program-related or patient-related crimes. The five-year exclusion was sustained.

C. Involuntary Manslaughter/Criminal Medical Negligence

The laws in each State define and establish the evidence required for various criminal acts. What typically distinguishes a criminal act from a civil act is *intent* and the *nature* of the harm. Just like civil actions, there are statute of limitations for criminal actions "to protect individuals from defending themselves against stale criminal charges, to prevent punishment for acts committed in the remote past, and to provide the accused with notice of the decision to prosecute and the general nature of the charge with sufficient promptness to allow the preparation of a defense."[65]

---

64 *In the case of: Burnette v. The Inspector General*, DAB No. CR496 (September 23, 1997).

65 *People v. Derbrugge*, 998 P.2d 43 (Co.App. 1999).

In *People v. Klvana*, Dr. Klvana was convicted of second degree murder, aiding and abetting the practice of medicine without license, conspiracy to practice medicine without a license, preparing fraudulent insurance claims, presenting false insurance claims, grand theft, and perjury.[66] Delores Doyle was a certified nurse assistant who worked with Dr. Klvana. In conjunction with this action, she was charged with three counts of murder, three alternative counts of involuntary manslaughter, five counts of practicing medicine without a license, one count of conspiracy to practice medicine without a license, 17 counts of preparing a fraudulent insurance claims, 9 counts of presenting false insurance claims, and one count of grand theft.

The actions brought against Dr. Klvana and CNA Doyle resulted from nine patient deaths. After the trial started, CNA Doyle entered a plea bargain under which she pled guilty to three counts of involuntary manslaughter, five counts of practicing medicine without a license, one count of conspiracy, and seven counts of insurance fraud.

Dr. Einaugler was convicted of reckless endangerment and second degree murder as a result of his failure to have a nursing home patient timely transferred to a hospital, resulting in the death of the patient.[67] Dr. Einaugler was employed in a nursing home when the resident was admitted. The resident had a peritoneal dialysis catheter which Dr. Einaugler thought was a gastrostomy feeding tube and directed that the resident be fed through the catheter. The resident received numerous feedings through the dialysis catheter before the mistake was discovered. When the mistake was reported to Dr. Einaugler and he became aware of the probable peritonitis which would be fatal if untreated, he did not order the resident transferred to the hospital for more than 10 hours. Upon admission to the hospital the resident was diagnosed with peritonitis which caused her death within a few days.

The evidence at trial was that Dr. Einaugler was aware of, and consciously disregarded, the substantial risk of serious physical injury to the resident by delaying her transfer to the hospital, and that his conduct constituted a gross deviation from the standard of care. In a criminal action, the standard for a jury is "beyond a reasonable doubt" while in a civil action the standard is "more likely than not." The jury concluded that there was sufficient evidence to establish reckless endangerment beyond a reasonable doubt based on evidence that Dr. Einaugler was aware of and consciously disregarded the substantial risk of severe physical injury to the resident by delaying her transfer to the hospital, and that his conduct was a gross deviation from the reasonable standard of care with

---

66 15 Cal.Rptr.2d 512 (Ca.App. 1992).

67 *People v. Einaugler*, 618 N.Y.S.2d 414 (N.Y.A.D. 1994), *habeas corpus denied in part, dismissed in part,* 918 F.Supp. 619 (E.D.N.Y. 1996).

his knowledge that peritonitis could be failure if untreated. There was also a charge of a misdemeanor of willful violation of the State health laws in that he willfully neglected the resident. As the court noted, the requisite mental state necessary for a conviction for violating a public health law requires more than *simple* negligence in the exercise of a clinical medical judgment, but rather requires proof of a *"willful"* failure to provide timely, consistent, safe, adequate, and appropriate treatment and/or care.[68]

A charge of negligent homicide was brought against a physician as the result of the death of an infant delivered at home.[69] To establish *negligent* homicide in Utah, the person must act with *criminal* negligence which results in the death of another person. Criminal negligence arises if the conduct is such that a person ought to be aware of a substantial and unjustifiable risk that the circumstances exist or the result will occur, and the failure to perceive the risk constitutes a gross deviation from the standard of care. The court discussed the difference between criminal negligence and civil negligence. As the court explained: "In situations where it is alleged that a medical doctor was negligent in the treatment of a patient, that doctor may be held civilly liable if the evidence establishes that it is *more likely* than not that the doctor's treatment failed below the appropriate standard of care. In contrast, a doctor may be held criminally liable only when the evidence establishes *beyond a reasonable doubt* that the doctor's treatment created a substantial and unjustifiable risk that the patient would die, that the doctor should have but failed to perceive this risk, and that the risk is of such a nature and degree that the failure to perceive it constitutes a gross deviation from the standard of care."[70] Evidence presented at trial was that Dr. Warden failed to examine the mother in the early stages of her labor and therefore did not diagnose the premature labor, take measures to stop the labor, or hospitalize her in anticipation of the premature birth. There was evidence that following delivery, Dr. Warden was aware that the infant had signs of respiratory distress syndrome. However, he told the parents that this symptom was a normal condition, stated that the baby did not need medical attention, and in fact, positioned the infant in a manner which masked the symptoms. Thus, the jury verdict of negligent homicide was upheld.

D. FALSIFYING HEALTH INFORMATION

In *State v. Whittle,* Barbara Whittle was the Director of Nursing at Royal Crest, a long term care facility in North Carolina.[71] Horace Keller, a resident at Royal

---

68 *Id.* at 416.

69 *State of Utah v. Warden*, 813 P.2d 1146 (Utah 1991).

70 *Id.* at 1151.

71 454 S.E.2d 688 (N.C. App. 1995).

Crest between August 31, 1989 and September 21, 1989, developed three decubiti on his heels and on his buttocks, which resulted in charges against Nurse Whittle. The charges included: falsification of Mr. Keller's admission report by documenting that these decubiti existed at a Stage IV level at the time he was admitted to Royal Crest; failure to implement procedures for the daily charting of unusual conditions, like decubiti; and failure to implement procedures for special skin care and care of decubiti. At trial, the State presented evidence that the decubiti did not exist at the time Mr. Keller was admitted to Royal Crest, and that Nurse Whittle altered Mr. Keller's admission records to so reflect. The State also alleged that Nurse Whittle acted unlawfully, willfully, and feloniously.

To find that Nurse Whittle committed the felony of malfeasance, the jury was instructed that the State must prove beyond a reasonable doubt that Nurse Whittle made a false entry, that Nurse Whittle knew the entry was false, and that Nurse Whittle willfully made the false entry regarding Horace Keller with the intent to deceive another person or corporation. To render a verdict that Nurse Whittle was guilty of a misdemeanor related to charting, the State had to prove beyond a reasonable doubt that Nurse Whittle, as Director of Nursing, willfully failed to cause the implementation of nursing procedures and policies for the daily charting of an unusual occurrence or acute episode relating to the development of decubiti on Horace Keller. For the jury to render a verdict that Nurse Whittle committed a misdemeanor related to special care, the State had to prove beyond a reasonable doubt that Nurse Whittle willfully failed to cause the implementation of nursing procedures for special skin care and decubiti care for Horace Keller.

The jury returned verdicts of guilty on the felony charge of malfeasance, and the two misdemeanor counts "willfully." But the court of appeals upheld the felony conviction.

REFERENCES

Albert, T., *Malpractice or Murder? Criminalization of Medical Errors Is a Troubling Trend,* American Medical News (October 22/29, 2001).

King, *Reduction of Likelihood Reformulation and Other Retrofitting of the Loss-of-a-Chance Doctrine,* 28 U. Mem. L. Rev. 491 (Winter 1998).

Kohn, L. T., Corrigan, J. M. & Donaldson, M. S., (editors), *To Err Is Human: Building a Safer Health System,* Institute of Medicine (2001).

Porter, K. A., *Dulaney v. Saint Alphonsus Regional Medical Center: Reconstructive Surgery For Plaintiff's Medical Nightmare—A Call For Reform of the Local Standard of Care,* 38 Idaho Law Review 597 (2002).

Rich, B. A., *A Prescription for the Pain—The Emerging Standard of Care for Pain Management,* 26 Wm. Mitchell L. Rev 1 (2000).

Rosenthal, M. & Schlesinger, *Not Afraid To Blame: The Neglected Role of Blame Attribution in Medical Consumerism and Some Implications For Health Policy,* 80 Milbank Q. 41 (2002).

Wampler, A.T., *Fly In The Buttermilk: Tennessee's Desire to Dispense With Layperson Common Sense and The Medical Malpractice Locality Rule,* 69 Tennessee Law Review 385 (Winter 2002).

CHAPTER 3

Professional Liability Insurance

SECTION 3-1: INSURANCE POLICY BASICS

Remember, nurses are human and human beings make errors: an incorrect dosage of medication is administered; a discoverable malignant breast mass goes undetected; an unrestrained elderly patient becomes confused and pulls out his endotracheal tube.

Although unintentional, the negligence of nurses causes harm to patients. The number of claims against nurses personally has dramatically increased and continues to increase. Sophisticated and specialized nursing standards of care are the norm. Lawsuits now expose nurses to damages equally comparable to damages awarded against physicians. Professional liability insurance provided protection for nurses and society when a patient is injured due to the nurse's failure to provide the acceptable standard of nursing care.

An uninsured or underinsured nurse is at financial risk. A judgment may be satisfied out of the nurse's personal assets. In some States, liens may be placed on property owned by the nurse, while other States permit wages to be garnished and future inheritances taken.

Regardless of the merit of a claim made against the nurse, legal steps must be taken by an attorney on behalf of the nurse. This requires money; if there is no professional liability insurance coverage available, the nurse personally pays.

Irrespective of whether a nurse has professional liability coverage purchased by an employer or personally, nurses must have a basic understanding of how the coverage works, what it covers, and the limitations. Being uninformed can be professionally, financially, and emotionally devastating.

Professional liability insurance is a contract in which one party (the "insurer") promises to assume the loss or liability imposed by law on another party (the "insured"), in exchange for a premium. In this contract, the insurer agrees to assume certain risks on behalf of the insured. The *insuring agreement* encompasses the basic promise of the insurer to act on behalf of the insured when a claim is made that is covered under the policy. This typically required the insurer to provide legal counsel and pay all legal-related expenses, and to pay damages in settlement or as awarded in a judgment against the insured.

The professionality liability insurance policy must be drafted specifically to cover a nurse's professional practice to afford maximum protection. It must provide coverage for *all* functions and acts undertaken by the nurse in *all* professional roles, such as involvement in peer review, quality determinations, and management roles.

The difficulty encountered most frequently by the courts in construing insurance policy provisions and coverage is to determine the intent of the parties as reflected by the language.

As Justice Holmes stated:

> A word is not a crystal, transparent and unchanged, it is the skin of a living though and may vary greatly in color and content according to the circumstances and the time in which it is used.[1]

Thus, courts interpret insurance contracts in light of their purpose and the specific facts to which the contracts are being applied. Any ambiguities are usually decided in the insured's benefit.[2]

SECTION 3-2: DUTIES AND OBLIGATIONS

Each professional liability insurance policy contains important conditions that must be complied with by the insured. Failure to comply with the conditions can create forfeiture of the policy and non-payment of claims.

A. Application

When completing an application for insurance, all information provided must be accurate and complete. If any portion of the insurance application is falsified and that information is relied upon by the insurer when considering the applicant, the policy may be void. This includes such items as stating a certificate is possessed when it is not, or lying about being previously named in a lawsuit.

---

1 *Towne v. Eisner*, 245 U.S. 418 (N.Y. 1918).

2 *Benham v. World Airways, Inc.*, 296 F.Supp. 813 (D.Hawaii 1969).

B. Notification

The insurer must be notified when the insured is aware that a lawsuit may arise based on the professional acts of the insured. In deciding what events need to be reported to an insurer, assess the facts of the situation. Then look at how the policy defines "claim." Typically, any occurrence where nursing judgment could be questioned or a bad outcome results must be reported. If a patient complaint is related to professional services rendered by or involving the insured, that may need to be reported. *Remember*, it is much better to err on the side of reporting what never becomes a claim than failing to report what subsequently results in a lawsuit. The insurer will promptly investigate the facts and circumstances to compile all the pertinent information. Witnesses may be located more easily and quickly, and their recollections will be more accurate. This results in a more intelligent evaluation of the potential liability and preparation of an adequate defense. The policy will state whether this notice requirement may be oral or must be written, and to whom it should be made.

If the insured fails to notify or delays notification, the insurer's obligation to provide coverage may be voided. Important factors in judging the reasonableness for the delay include:

1. Length of delay in giving notice;
2. Reasons for the delay; and
3. Probable effect of the delay on the insurer.

If an insurer fails to honor a claim because of alleged late notice, and the insured wishes to challenge that refusal, an action seeking a declaratory judgment may be brought asking a court to determine the reasonableness of the insurer's position. The court will also determine the obligations of the insurer to the insured under the terms of the insurance policy. Such an action was initiated by St. Louis University against its insurer for a mistake in notification.[3] Lexington Insurance Company issued the professional liability insurance policy to St. Louis University for claims made from July 1, 1990–July 1, 1991. On May 20, 1991, a patient sued the University for malpractice allegedly committed in 1979. In a report submitted to the insurance company, St. Louis University mistakenly listed the claim date as 1979 rather than 1991. Because this was a claims-made policy the timeliness of the notice is not merely related to the insured's duty to cooperate; rather, it defines the limits of the insurer's obligation. "A claims-made policy allows the insurer to more accurately fix its reserves for future liabilities and compute premiums with greater certainty."[4]

---

3 *Lexington Insurance Company v. St. Louis University*, 88 F.3d 632 (8th Cir. 1996).

4 *Id.* at 1.

The court noted that many states, including Missouri, have adopted regulations prohibiting unfair insurance claims settlement practices. Generally, an insurer cannot deny a claim based upon the failure of the insured to submit a written notice of the loss within a specified time, unless the failure operates to prejudice the rights of the insurer. Therefore, the insurer need not prove prejudice to avoid coverage under a claims-made policy if the claim was not reported until after the policy expired. The court therefore concluded that as a matter of law there was no coverage because timely reporting of claims to the insurer under a claims-made policy is an essential part of the contract.

When an insured has more than one insurance policy applicable to a claim, notification must be made to all insurers. It then becomes the obligation of the insurance companies to resolve among themselves as to who pays for what.

When an insured knows a lawsuit has been filed with the insured as a named defendant or whose negligence is being attributed to a third party, the insurer must be notified immediately. There are legal requirements to be taken, and there are time constraints imposed by law when a lawsuit is filed.

C. Duty to Defend

The insurer's duty to defend the insured is the primary focus of the protection afforded and by the professional liability insurance policy. The insurer is obligated to arrange for and pay legal expenses and costs to defend claims brought against the insured. These expenses and costs are not limited by or included in the policy limits, unless specifically set forth as such in the insurance contract.

Whether there is a duty to defend the insured is determined by the allegations against the insured and whether they fall under the coverage provided by the policy. Any allegations within the policy terms triggers the insurer's duty, regardless of the truth of falsity of the allegations. If the facts or allegations are ambiguous, the insurer must still defend. Until such time as the claims are determined to be outside the policy coverage, the duty of the insurer continues.

D. Appointment of Legal Counsel

The insurer hires and designates legal counsel to represent the insured. Because the insured is entitled to *effective* legal representation, if the insured questions the adequacy of legal services being rendered, the insured has a right to notify the insurer of these concerns and request different legal counsel.

Because nurses are infrequently (thankfully) involved in lawsuits, they typically don't know what they should expect from or be entitled to from AN attorney. It is expected that the attorney consult regularly with the nurse to investigate the allegations and determine the defense. The nurse may be requested to obtain clinical information and resources, review health information, prepare for and attend depositions, and identify experts. In return, the nurse has the right to expect a certain level of competency from the attorney.

These expectations are well stated by Tom Fisher, a prestigious and wise attorney at Shughart, Thomson & Kilroy:

1. A lawyer's three core standards: analysis; research; communication (ARC).
2. When a lawyer calls or writes, immediately call that lawyer back.
3. Keep your client informed (for lots of reasons).
4. Settle the "dogs" early and save your client's money.
5. Do not delegate what you have never done.
6. Believe in your client's case. If you don't, no one else will.
7. Be honest when dealing with judges, lawyers, and clients. Credibility is your currency and it will pay dividends in the long run.
8. When arguing a legal point, don't just say what the law is; say why the law makes sense.
9. Understand the weaknesses of your case. Don't ignore them because the other side won't.
10. If you do not thoroughly prepare your case, you will not achieve the best result.
11. Take one or more vacations every year. Life is short and vacation gives prospective.[5]

Ethical issues may confront an attorney who represents the insured. The attorney, although obligated to the insured who is the attorney's client, in effect, is being paid by and therefore also acting on behalf of the insurer. This requires the attorney to exercise a high duty of care to both clients.

The attorney may learn facts from the insured that are unknown to the insurer, which create questions of whether the insurer is obligated to defend the insured under the policy. For example, coverage may not apply if the insured violated a law. Thus, if an allegation against the insured is that of practicing beyond the parameters of the Nurse Practice Act, and the attorney's investigation confirms this happened, the attorney arguably has a duty to relate those findings to the insurer. In turn, the insurer could then refuse to defend the insured under the conditions of the policy. Any nurse who anticipates such a potential problem should consult a private attorney.

---

5 Tom Fisher, *11 Commandments for the Practice of Law,* STK Insider (January 10, 2003). A special thanks to Tom for allowing me to share his wisdom with others.

E. Good Faith

A professional liability insurance policy imposes an implied covenant of good faith and fairness on both the insurer and insured. Each party consents to refrain from acts or omissions that could prevent the other from receiving any benefits of the contract. Violation of this good faith agreement could expose a party to an action for breach of contract and damages.

If an insurer acts in bad faith, the insured may be covered for any expenses incurred, and perhaps even entitled to punitive or other damages for emotional distress. Bad faith is not simply a bad judgment but implies the conscious doing of a wrong with the nature of fraud. Examples of bad faith include rejecting the advice of legal counsel or statements that there is little or nothing to lose by refusing to settle.

Some courts distinguish between bad faith and negligence when determining liability of an insurer. Insurers are liable for both bad faith as well as negligence. Examples of negligence on behalf of an insurer include: (a) not properly conducting the defense of a case; (b) failing to carefully and prudently investigate the facts and interview witnesses; (c) failing to present competent and material evidence at trial; or (d) making improper stipulations.

F. Appeals

The terms of the professional liability insurance policy will dictate the obligation of the insurer to appeal an adverse judgment awarded against an insured. There is no independent duty imposed upon the insurer to proceed with an appeal. Generally the agreement to defend provided by the insurance contract does not create an obligation for the insurer to file or pay for an appeal. However, failure to appeal has been grounds for an improperly conducted defense by an insurer.

SECTION 3-3: EXCLUSIONS AND LIMITATIONS

Every professional liability insurance policy has defined exclusions and limitations where the policy is not effective.

A. Criminal Actions

If the allegation is that the insured violated a criminal statute or ordinance, coverage is not extended as criminal acts are not within the scope of the insuring clause.

B. Intentional Torts

Other acts that are "criminal" in nature may be excluded under the policy and yet potentially committed by nurses, such as assault and battery, defamation and false imprisonment. These are intentional torts. These may arise from failure to obtain consent or placing an individual in restraints without sufficient cause. However, most policies will provide coverage for these acts unless there is evidence of any willful or specific intent to do harm.

There's no general rule as to what constitutes an "intentional tort" within the context of an insurance contract. Two factors important in determining whether an intentional tort comes within the exclusionary clause of the policy are:

1. The legal meaning attributed by the court to the exclusionary clause; and
2. The application of the court-defined clause to the particular facts in the case.

The general consensus is that an injury is intentional if the insured acted with the specific intent to cause harm to a certain third party.

Courts have held coverage is applicable where the allegations involve professional nursing services rendered or incidents directly connected with the nurse's practice. A question of coverage may arise for statements made about a colleague's incompetency or as a member of a professional board or hospital committee.

C. Practicing Beyond Nurse Practice Act

There is no beyond insurance coverage for a nurse who exceeds the scope of a State Nurse Practice Act or license. Coverage is for losses incurred from acts or omissions arising out of the practice of *nursing*. If allegations of practicing medicine are asserted against the insured, the insurer may not defend those claims, or refuse to pay any settlement or judgment against the insured.

D. Punitive Damages

As a matter of public policy, professional liability insurance policies exclude coverage for punitive damages awarded against an insured. Punitive damages are rendered to punish actions that involve actual malice or reckless disregard for another. They are to deter such actions in the future. These are damages over and above those damages awarded to compensate actual injury. If an insurance policy covers punitive damages, how will the insured be punished or deterred?

There has been movement away from the public argument against providing insurance to cover punitive damages. The courts are split, with the majority holding that where the policy provisions make no distinction between actual and punitive damages, the contract terms encompass liability for punitive damages. Even those jurisdictions that hold public policy precludes insurance coverage

43

for punitive damages still impose a duty on the insurer to defend where allegations in the complaint comingle claims for compensatory and punitive damages.

To decide the insurer's obligation to pay punitive damages, courts examine closely the language of the insurance contract. If the policy provides payment of "all sums which the insured shall become legally obligated to pay as damages," some courts have held insurers liable for punitive damages as they are damages which the insured is "legally obligated to pay." More courts require the insurer to expressly exclude punitive damages from coverage if that is the intent. Public policy requires full performance of a contract between an insurer and insured, and where there are ambiguities or mere generalities these are frequently resolved to the benefit of the insured.

SECTION 3-4: SETTLEMENT

The implications and significance of settling claims is interpreted differently. To the insured, settlement represents an admission of wrongdoing. While that may be one reason for settlement, many other reasons result in a decision to settle: (a) the insurer's evaluation of the allegations of negligence may differ from the insured's and raise some doubt concerning a successful defense; (b) the uncertainties of trial by jury often convince the insurer that the best odds are with settlement; (c) early on after a claim is made, the patient may be willing to settle for a small amount of money; and (d) recognizing that defense costs may exceed the settlement, the insurer's business sense will dictate that decision. Insurers prefer to fight non-meritorious claims, but also must balance the economics of the situation. Insurers have witnessed cases which they believed to be very defensible and yet verdicts are awarded to the plaintiffs.

An insurer has a fiduciary duty to an insured. This creates a relationship and obligation of trust and good faith, so the insured can rely upon the integrity and fidelity of the insurer who occupies this position of confidence. As such, the insurer has an affirmative duty to explore settlement possibilities and to initiate negotiations of settlement for policy limits when in the best interest of the insured.

In most professional liability insurance policies, the insurer reserves the right to compromise or settle claims or lawsuits. The terms of the insurance policy will dictate whether the insurer may settle a claim without the consent of the insured. If the insurance policy fails to include any clause regarding settlement, the insurer retains sole authority to make such decisions.

If an insurer refuses to accept a reasonable settlement offer, it may be liable for the full judgment rendered against the insured, even where the policy coverage limits are exceeded. In determining whether an insurer has acted appropriately in rejecting a settlement offer, such factors will be considered as: (a) has the insurer taken into account the interest of the insured and given equal consideration to those interests and its own; (b) was a realistic evaluation of the case and the potential magnitude of an award made by the insurer; (c) did the insurer properly investigate the circumstances of the claim; (d) was reasonable consideration given by the insured to the seriousness of the injuries involved.

Some professional liability insurance policies allow the insured the right to reject any settlement decision proposed by the insurer. However, if the insured refuses to accept the proposed settlement and a judgment is ultimately rendered against the insured, it is possible that the insurer's liability will be limited to the settlement offer. That should be specified in the policy.

However, where the insurer fails to provide the insurer the option of accepting or rejecting a settlement offer, that may constitute a breach of the contract. In that event, the insurer becomes liable for any damages resulting therefrom, including any damages exceeding the policy limits.

SECTION 3-5: TYPES OF POLICIES

The three general types of professional liability insurance policies are: claims-made; occurrence; and claims-paid. The policies differ by the coverage period during which time the insurer agrees to assume risks on behalf of the insured. The effectiveness of the insurance policy is limited to this specific time period and will not apply to acts occurring outside those dates.

A. Claims-Made

Claims-made policies cover claims reported while the policy is in force. These protect the insured for professional services rendered either during the policy period or prior thereto, provided the *claim* is reported during the policy's effective dates.

The term "claim" is generally very broadly defined to include lawsuits, allegations by a patient or an attorney, notice received from a dissatisfied patient, or awareness by the insured of potential harm to a patient from personal negligence. Know how the insurance policy defines claim! A lawsuit doesn't have to be filed for an incident to be covered by a claims-made policy. Notice must be given to the insurer during the policy period to obtain coverage for a lawsuit filed in the future.

Under a claims-made policy, if a nurse administers an injection to a patient and strikes the sciatic nerve, causing paralysis, notify the insurer immediately because this is a potential lawsuit. If an alleged act of negligence occurs during the period of coverage but notice is not given to the insurer within that time, the insurer can deny coverage if a lawsuit is filed in the future.

45

B. Occurrence

An *occurrence* policy provides protection for *all acts or omissions* that occur *during* the policy period. Coverage extends to any claims that result, even if not reported until after the termination of that policy period. Thus, under an occurrence policy, an alleged act of negligence by the insured can occur within the policy period but neither the insured nor the insurer are notified or made aware of the allegation until several years later.

The potential conflict with an occurrence policy is when an injury results from treatment that extends both within and outside the policy period. Whether there is coverage provided under the insurance policy may be questioned. The "occurrence" within the context of the liability policy refers to when the damage occurred rather than when the negligent act or omission caused the damage. With progressive diseases, "occurrence" is clearly inherently ambiguous. If the allegation against the nurse is failure to refer a patient with a diagnosis of cancer, whom the nurse treats over a period of years, when was the "occurrence?"

If the insurer questions its duty to provide coverage because of the timing of the occurrence, an action may be brought before a court either by the insurer or the insured to determine whether coverage is available.

C. Claims-Paid

A variation of claims-made policies are *claims-paid* policies. They typically provide a cheaper but more restrictive form of claims-made policies. Claims must be made *and* paid during the policy period: (1) the medical treatment and injury gave rise to the claim during policy; (2) the claim was asserted against the insured and reported to the insurer; and (3) the claim was paid. Therefore, if a claims-paid policy is purchased for the year 1990, renewed for the year 1991, a claim that is made and reported in 1990 and is paid in 1991 is covered. However, if the claims-paid policy wasn't renewed for 1991, the claim would not be paid under the coverage purchased in 1990.

Premiums for claims-paid policies may be significantly lower upfront, but tail coverage or extended reporting endorsements that would need to be purchase are significantly higher. The differences in costs are due to the ability of the insurer to plan short-term and shift the cost from the base premium to the extended coverage.

Some claims-paid policies may offer the insured free or lost-cost tail coverage upon disability, retirement, or death. For insured who intends to remain with the same insurer for the course of their professional careers may benefit from claims-paid policies.

SECTION 3-6: PURCHASING A POLICY

A. Personal Policy: Pros and Cons

Nurses are seldom well informed regarding the extent to which they are afforded protection under an employer's professional liability insurance policy. An employer's policy covers actions of the nurse employee performed within the scope of employment. Thus, the insurer for the employer can deny coverage for actions performed outside the scope of the job description or employment setting,

Employers may seek indemnification against employees for damages they must pay because of acts or omissions by employees. It would produce chilling effects in employer-employee relationships, creating adversarial environments that are not conducive to the necessary cohesive and professional working relationship between employees and their employers.

Nurses may be sued for actions that occur outside of their employment and are obviously not covered by their employers' policies. Good Samaritan Laws were enacted to provide legal immunity to persons who assist in medical emergencies, but usually provide *absolute* immunity against claims or lawsuits; actions that are grossly negligent or malicious or not immune from liability. Nursing-related services volunteered at health fairs or other community activities are subject to lawsuits. Even offering advice to a neighbor exposes the nurse to a potential lawsuit for which an employer policy is totally useless.

Although an argument frequently heard is that having a personal insurance policy invites more lawsuits or larger judgments, the reality is that nurses are sued without knowledge of the presence or absence of insurance. In most States juries are not even permitted to know whether insurance is involved. If an action is filed against a nurse without any reasonable belief that the nurse was negligent, solely because of awareness that liability insurance is available, that attorney is subject to a malicious prosecution action by the nurse. Attorneys do not randomly name defendants in lawsuits.

Whether to purchase a personal professional liability insurance policy is a personal decision for the nurse. Take into consideration factors such as: involvement in professional activities outside of the employment setting; personal assets, both current and future inheritances; advanced nurse practice activities engaged in; for coverage provided by an employer, the type of policy, extent of coverage when no longer employed there, the financial viability of the employer, and the policy limits; potential for lawsuits in nursing practice area; the magnitude of awards rendered in that area of nursing; and what personally is reassuring.

B. Policy Limits

A professional liability insurance policy limits the amounts paid on behalf of the insured. Payment includes compensable damages for any injuries directly and proximately resulting and causing physical damages, financial damages, and/or emotional damages.

The insurer is only liable for damages totaling set maximum dollar amounts as provided in the policy. Those limits are usually stated as $X/$Y, with $X representing the dollar amount per occurrence or claim, and $Y representing the aggregate dollar amount per the policy period. The limits of liability per each claim apply regardless of the number of persons who sustain injury or the number of claims made for losses resulting from any one occurrence.

If the policy limits are $1,000,000/$3,000,000, the insured has $1,000,000 available to satisfy a judgment or settlement rendered as a result of any one occurrence causing injuries. If a wife sustains injury resulting from the nurse's negligence, and her husband claims loss of consortium, the maximum amount of money available to both the husband and wife is $1,000,000.

The aggregate dollar amount, $3,000,000, is the total limit of the insurer's liability for all settlements and judgments rendered against the insured during the coverage period of the policy. There is no limit on the number of lawsuits against which the insurer will defend the insured during the policy period; rather, the only limit is on the total amount of money to be paid as a result of all claims.

C. Which Policy Is Best

While one type of policy is not particularly better than the other, the issue with claims-made and claims-paid policies is that when the insured retires or leaves the practice of nursing, *or* changes coverage to an occurrence policy, there is no coverage for claims yet to be asserted for prior acts or omissions. To protect the insured, insurance companies offer a "Reporting Endorsement" or "Tail Coverage Policy" that preserves the coverage offered under the prior claims-made policy. However, these tend to be somewhat expensive, and the insured must remember that a supplemental policy is necessary to extend any claims-made or claims-paid policy.

REFERENCES

American Medical Association, *The Guide to Medical Professional Liability Insurance* (1991).

Blumenreich, G.A., *Who Does Your Lawyer Represent?* 59 AANA Journal 390 (Oct. 1991).

Henry, P.F., *Overview of MalPractice Insurance.* 5 Nurse Practitioner Forum 4 (March 1994).

Kemmy, J., *Professional Liability Insurance Coverage for Perioperative Nurses.* 56 AORN Journal 526 (Sept. 1992).

Kane, Leslie, *Are There Gaps In Your Malpractice Coverage?* 227 Medical Economics (March 23, 1998).

CHAPTER 4

Lawsuit Anatomy

SECTION 4-1: INTRODUCTION

Litigation threatens and creates intense fear in nurses. With the overwhelming civil and criminal litigious climate, adversarial relationships have resulted. Nurses are being sued not only by patients, but also by Federal government agencies, State nursing regulatory agencies, and prosecutors. Penalties imposed may be fines, prison terms, punitive damages, and loss of nursing license.

The early beginnings of medico-legal practice focused on forensic medicine, examining the cause of death to determine whether criminal charges should be filed. When an individual died from a disease, the person charged was frequently the physician. This occurred as early as 900 A.D. Even then, experts would testify at trial regarding the findings of autopsy or other aspects surrounding the death.

The study of forensic medicine precipitated writings and teachings and remained the primary legal concern in medicine for approximately four hundred years. The physician's performance was compared with that of other physicians in the same community. In the fourteenth century in England, surgical malpractice suits appeared in legal documents. However, medical aspects of the law developed slowly in the United States, with the first lectures and writings and legal actions for malpractice not occurring until the nineteenth century.

Significant transitions have affected the legal status of nurses. In large, these have been influenced and shaped by societal movements. The status of nurses has directly correlated with the position women occupy within society.

Nurses are trying to "help" patients with reimbursement so patients get the care deemed necessary. Tactics include exaggerating the severity of symptoms, manipulating billing diagnoses, and falsifying information and signatures.

51

Inappropriately coding diagnoses or services or falsely certifying the need for a certain level of care is *fraud*. If these acts are done *intentionally*, they are criminal. Even if specific intent is not shown, civil fraud can be proven if conduct is with "reckless disregard" or "deliberate ignorance."

All States have required reporting laws, such as for child and elder abuse and neglect, communicable diseases, criminally caused wounds, and disease registries. Many States require a nurse to report to the State nursing regulatory agency knowledge that another nurse violated the Nurse Practice Act. Failure to report will trigger criminal prosecution or licensure investigation.

A study of lawsuits that were filed from 1988 through 1993 found that in 747 cases, nursing negligence in hospitals caused or contributed to negative patient outcomes and resulted in a plaintiff's verdict or settlement.[1] 219 patients died due to nursing negligence. Causes for these deaths included: (a) inadequate communication by a nurse to a physician: 76 deaths; (b) inadequate patient assessment: 46 deaths; (c) medication administration errors: 42 deaths; (d) inadequate nursing intervention: 17 deaths; (e) inadequate care: 21 deaths; (f) unsafe environment: 7 deaths; (g) inadequate infection control: 3 deaths; and (h) improper use of equipment and products: 7 deaths.

In a 2001 Gallup poll, nurses were perceived as No. 1 by the public in honesty compared to other professions such a pharmacists (No. 2), veterinarians (No. 3), and physicians (No. 4). The were also ranked as No. 1 in ethical behavior which is the same rating received by the clergy.[2]

Because nurses are unfamiliar with legal actions, there is an inherent discomfort when called upon to participate in them. Legal proceedings often create an air of intimidation that only adds to the anxiety. Nurses are frequently involved in legal actions, fortunately more often as witnesses than as defendants. It is important that the nurse understand the legal process and develop skills to make the nurse as effective as possible.

SECTION 4-2: INITIATION OF LAWSUIT

A. Parties and Where Filed

A lawsuit is initiated by the filing of a document referred to as a petition or complaint. This document identifies all parties to the action, both plaintiffs and defendants. "Plaintiffs" are those persons who are bringing the lawsuit; the "defendants" are the individuals being sued.

---

1 Janet Pitts Beckman, *Nursing Negligence* (1st Edition 1996).

2 S. Williams, *Split Decisions: Nursing Profession Ranks Low in Desirability of Publics' High Regard for Nurses,* Nurses Week (April 16, 2001); L. Joseph and A. Lewis, *Who Has the Highest Ethics*, USA Today 1A June 4, 2004).

Plaintiffs in a malpractice action include the injured patient and any family members who allege that they have been damages due to the patient's injury. All of those parties must bring their action in one lawsuit. The courts do not allow separate lawsuits to be filed by the patient, spouse, and children.

The defendants in a lawsuit include individual health care providers, supervisory or administrative personnel, and their employers. All potential defendants in an action must also be sued in the same lawsuit.

Lawsuits may be filed in either State or Federal court, depending upon where the parties reside. Within a State, they have to be filed in the county either where the parties reside or where the cause of action occurred.

In a malpractice action, all four elements that must be proven by the plaintiffs must be included in the petition/complaint: duty; negligence/malpractice; causation of an injury; and damages. If any of these elements is missing, a motion will be filed to dismiss the lawsuit because it "fails to state a cause of action."

B. Answer and Defenses

In response to the petition/complaint, each defendant files a document referred to as an "answer." This admits or denies the allegations contained in the petition/complaint and includes any available defenses. For example, malpractice actions must be brought within the State's statute of limitations. If on the face of the petition/complaint the lawsuit is being filed beyond the appropriate statute of limitations, that is asserted as a defense.

The answer must be filed with the court within a set time frame. The failure to do so will result in the plaintiff being awarded a judgment by default, meaning the plaintiff prevails. Thus, it is extremely important to immediately notify your professional liability insurance carrier if you are served with a lawsuit.

A defense to the petition/complaint may be statutory immunity. This is where either a Federal or State law provides that under defined circumstances certain people may be immune from being sued and/or immune from liability. For example, the Federal Health Care Quality Improvement Act (HCQIA) was enacted in 1986 to provide peer review participants with qualified immunity. The scope of this immunity has been extended for *all* peer review participants, including non-physicians.[3] The HCQIA creates a rebuttal presumption of immunity, which forces the plaintiff to prove that the defendants failed to comply with the relevant standards. This immunity has been upheld in the majority of peer review cases.

---

3 *Meyers v. Columbia/HCA Healthcare Corporation*, 341 F.3d 461 (6th Cir. 2003).

C. Discovery

Discovery is the process where the attorneys seek information to learn the facts and opinions about the case. States tend to have very liberal discovery rules that encourage the open exchange of information. This facilitates the dismissal of non-meritorious claims or settlement where there is obvious liability.

The discovery process includes interrogatories, requests for production of documents, and depositions. Interrogatories are questions that are exchanged between the parties whereby basic information is obtained. These allow the parties to learn the general contentions being made and to begin gathering pertinent information needed to proceed with the lawsuit.

The request for production of documents requires the parties to produce documents that are requested by the other side. For example, plaintiffs are asked to produce any calendars maintained during the time at issue, medical bills and expenses paid, evidence of lost wages, and photographs that show the claimed injury. Defendants may be asked to produce documents such as: the health care facility's bylaws, policies, procedures, protocols, critical paths, clinical practice guidelines, and standards of care; personnel files of defendant employees; a listing of continuing education programs offered and who attended at the health care facility; patient acuity logs; and staffing records.

After initial information is learned through interrogatories and the request for production of documents, the next step is to proceed with depositions. Usually the depositions of the parties are taken first, followed by depositions of factual witnesses. These are people who may have knowledge of the events that occurred or who have been personal health care providers for the injured patient. The final depositions include those of the expert witnesses, those individuals who will be testifying on behalf of plaintiffs and defendants at trial.

The discovery process can take anywhere from a year up to five years or even more, depending upon the number of parties in the action and the complexity of the alleged claims. At the conclusion of discovery is typically where the parties will consider settlement.

D. Trial

At trial, the first step is selecting a jury. A panel of potential jurors are questioned by the court and/or the attorneys for the plaintiffs and defendants. This process is called "voir dire" which means "to speak the truth." The purpose is to select a jury who will fairly and impartially hear the evidence in the case and decide the facts. The number of jurors selected depends on State law, but is usually twelve. If it is anticipated that the trial will be lengthy, one or two alternates may also be selected who will sit with the jury throughout the trial.

After the jury is selected, opening statements are given by the attorneys. Throughout the trial, the attorney for the plaintiffs always goes first because the plaintiffs have the burden of proof. The plaintiffs must present sufficient evidence of each element to allow the case to be ultimately decided by the jury. Therefore, the plaintiffs' attorney gives an opening statement followed by the defendants' attorneys giving opening statements. The purpose of the opening statements is to provide the jury with a framework for the evidence and witness testimony. It gives the jury a road map as to what the lawsuit is all about and how it will proceed.

The next step in the trial is to present the evidence through witnesses and exhibits. The plaintiffs' attorney begins by presenting the case on behalf of the plaintiffs. Witnesses are called who testify under oath as to the facts and opinions pertaining to the issues. When the plaintiffs' attorney calls a witness, *direct examination* is performed by the plaintiffs' attorney. The defendants' attorneys then have the opportunity to *cross-examine* the witness at that time. After the plaintiffs' attorney has put on all of the evidence on behalf of plaintiffs, the plaintiffs rest. The defendants then proceed to put on their case. At the conclusion of all of defendants' evidence, the plaintiffs' attorney may be allowed to put on *rebuttal* evidence to counter any new evidence that was presented during the defendants' case.

Jury instructions are then read by the judge to the jurors which instruct the jury how to apply the law once they decide the facts in the case. The charge to the jury is to decide what facts they believe to be true depending upon the credibility of the witnesses and other evidence. They are then instructed that if they find certain things to be true, the law must be specifically applied as set forth in the instructions. Jurors use the jury instructions during deliberation. The jury instructions include the verdict form that must be completed by the jury.

The final step in the trial are closing arguments. As it implies, this is an opportunity for the attorneys to argue their case to point out deficiencies in the other's case, attack the credibility of witnesses, and highlight the strong aspects of their own case. Again, the plaintiffs' attorney proceeds first with closing argument, followed by defendants' attorneys, and then plaintiffs' attorney gets the final word. Closing arguments tend to be very emotional. Both sides are making an appeal to the jury to decide the case in their favor.

After the closing arguments, the jury is taken to the deliberation room. They are permitted to take any exhibits that were introduced at trial. The jury elects a foreperson who controls the jury deliberations. The jurors are not permitted to talk to anyone, including the judge, during this process. If the jury has a question, it is sent in a written communication to the judge, who reads it and shows it to the attorneys. Very seldom can a jury question be answered.

Once a jury has reached its verdict, the jurors return to the courtroom and the verdict is given to the judge. The judge reads the verdict and enters the ruling of the court to either accept or refuse the verdict. The trial is then over.

The judge may permit the attorneys to talk with the jurors following the conclusion of the trial. However, jurors are not compelled to talk with anyone. The dialogue with the jurors can provide important feedback to the attorneys. They have an opportunity to find out what evidence the jurors considered the most credible or least credible, how they were affected by certain witnesses, what tactics may have been successful or unsuccessful, and other important aspects of the trial that may have been factors in how the verdict was rendered.

If a judgment is awarded against the defendants, it is first satisfied from any insurance assets. Only after insurance assets are exhausted will the plaintiffs proceed against the personal assets of the defendants. State laws vary as to what personal assets can be obtained to satisfy a judgment.

SECTION 4-3: DEPOSITIONS

Depositions are the opportunity for the attorneys to question parties and witnesses. During depositions, other witnesses may be identified. They also serve to preserve testimony as deposition transcripts may be used at trial under certain circumstances. An additional value is to evaluate a witness's effectiveness, credibility, demeanor, and appearance as those are also important considerations for the jury.

At a deposition, the attorneys for all parties are present and frequently the parties are also present. A court reporter records verbatim everything that is said during the proceeding and creates a transcript.

The person being deposed (who is being asked the questions) is the deponent. An attorney should always be present to provide protection for the deponent, such as advising the deponent when questions are not legally required to be answered or that breach any confidentialities or privileges, and to make legal objections for a judge to rule upon before the deposition testimony may be used at trial. The attorney is also a resource person for the deponent during the proceeding if any questions arise.

Although depositions are not conducted in the formality of a courtroom nor is a judge present, they are extremely important. The testimony rendered at a deposition may determine whether an action will be pursued, settled, or dismissed. Sufficient time must be spent by the deponent and attorney preparing for the deposition.

Before the deposition review relevant documents, especially health information, so they are familiar. Other documents, such as deposition transcripts, medical articles and texts, and opinions of expert witnesses are beneficial for the deponent to review. While documents may be referred to during a deposition, familiarity with them will enhance the accuracy and effectiveness of the deponent's testimony and allow the deposition to proceed with greater ease.

Understand the purpose of the deposition as this will identify the focus of the deponent's testimony. While it may be helpful for factual witnesses to meet together to discuss the events being investigated to stimulate recall in one another of facts that are not documented, this should *only* be done with an attorney present to protect discovery of those conversations and to avoid falsifying recollections.

During depositions minimize distractions. Make arrangements for telephone calls or beepers to be handled by someone else. If the deposition is in an unfamiliar setting, arrive early to familiarize yourself and become comfortable. Prior to beginning, spend a few minutes reviewing with your attorney deposition guidelines and any documents brought by you to the proceeding.

A court reporter takes down everything that is said, so allow the questioning attorney to complete the question before answering to prevent two people from talking at the same time. Speak clearly, avoid non-verbal answers and slang words, or other words that may not be clearly understood in the transcript.

The format of a deposition is for an attorney to ask a specific question to which the deponent gives an equally specific answer. The most important rule: listen carefully to the question! It is human nature to anticipate what is going to be asked or to volunteer more information than is being requested (especially by nurses!).

It is not the deponent's responsibility to divulge information. If a question is unclear, ambiguous, or compound, ask the attorney to explain what is meant or define terms before answering the question. Don't personally attempt to clarify the question or assume what it means.

Because nurses are constantly educating patients and other health care providers, they easily assume the role of educating attorneys. However, depositions are not the appropriate place to be helpful when in an adversarial position with the questioning attorney.

Don't guess or speculate if unsure of an answer. Before answering a question, take time to think about it and formulate your answer. "I don't recall or remember at this time" and "I don't know" are entirely appropriate and may be the best answers. If being questioned about events that occurred several years ago, it is highly unlikely that all facts are going to be recalled or known. Any answer that is rendered in a deposition, regardless of the degree of speculation, in effect becomes a fact at the time of trial.

Above all, *always tell the truth*. A lie totally destroys your credibility and effectiveness, and creates an inference of dishonesty about other testimony rendered. If there is an obvious error, don't cover it up or argue over some technical aspect. On the other hand, don't fall into the trap of agreeing with an attorney that an action was an error if that is a disputed issue in the lawsuit.

Be fair and accurate about events; avoid exaggerating. Watch against rendering opinions outside your area of expertise. Any opinions rendered may be interpreted as being expert opinions and used against other parties. Don't render an opinion if it is based upon false or insufficient information. If the attorney presents a set of hypothetical facts, make certain that there is enough information for a reasonable opinion to be rendered.

In answering questions, be brief and specific. If the question calls for a simple "yes" or "no", then that is the complete answer. Make the attorney follow-up with additional questions if more information is wanted. If a question is very broad and calls for an extensive narrative answer, ask the attorney to break down the question so that it can be specifically answered.

Attorneys may make very oversimplified and broad statements that are seemingly harmless but then lead to a damaging conclusion. These are sometimes phrased as leading questions which, in effect, allow the attorney to do the testifying with the deponent only agreeing or disagreeing. The purpose of the deposition is for the *deponent* to give personal testimony, not the *attorney*. Watch for generalizations as they often can lead to damaging testimony, especially where they are not applicable to the specifics of the particular case or proceeding.

Because the deposition transcript can be read to the jury, avoid angry, sarcastic, or flippant remarks, or inappropriate language. If you become angry or upset, take a break to avoid making remarks on the record. Remember, you as the *deponent control* the deposition! Take breaks when you need to.

After answering a question, don't hedge your answer. Be firm and assertive; do not change answers. If the attorney attempts to force recall or suggest alternate answers, merely restate the answer previously given.

Watch for silence after an answer; it may trigger the deponent to provide additional information. Guard against doing that.

During a deposition, the attorney acting on the deponent's behalf may object to questions. The purposes for these objections: (1) legally attorneys are required to preserve questions to be ruled on by the judge prior to testimony being read at trial; and (2) they alert the deponent to problematic questions. Listen to the objections as they may point out deficiencies in the question that are important to consider before rendering an answer. The objection may be that the question is calling for information that is privileged and therefore the question does not have to be answered. Unless instructed not to answer a question, the deponent must render some response, even if it is that the question cannot be answered.

If the deponent has talked with other persons about the case, the questioning attorney has the right to discover who those persons are. Unless those discussions have included an attorney, the names of those people must be disclosed as well as the general nature of those discussions. An inference can be made that testimony was jointly agreed upon and is not the independent testimony of the deponent.

Experts and certain factual witnesses will be compensated for their time and expenses. This may be asked by the attorney so be prepared to appropriately answer. Being paid a reasonable fee doesn't adversely affect the credibility of the deponent's testimony.

Prior to concluding the proceeding, if any wrong answers were given or areas need to be clarified, those should be discussed with your attorney. Many times it is beneficial to clarify the record immediately rather than do it at a later date.

At the conclusion of the deposition, the deponent will be asked what should be done with the prepared transcript. Every deponent has the right to review the final transcript. The options of the deponent are:

1. Require the court reporter to appear in person, present the transcript to the deponent, record any corrections to the deponent's testimony, and notarize the deponent's signature to approve the transcript contents.
2. Waive formal presentation by the reporter, but have the transcript sent to the deponent or the deponent's attorney for the deponent to review and make any corrections, sign before any Notary Public, and return to the reporter or attorney.
3. Waive all of the above and accept the accuracy of the contents.

Option 2 is recommended. Since the deposition transcript needs to conform with testimony at trial or it may be used in lieu of trial testimony, any discrepancies need to be identified and corrected as soon as possible.

SECTION 4-4: EXPERT WITNESSES

To prove that a nurse committed malpractice there must be evidence of the standard of care expected of the nurse and how the nurse failed to meet that standard. Historically this has required testimony of a person designated and qualified as an expert witness. However, now the standard of care and deviation from it can be proved by documents that clearly reflect expected standards and testimony from the nurse of how that standard wasn't met.

An expert witness is an individual who is qualified by education, experience, employment, publications, or research to render an opinion because the jury is confronted with an area that is so technical and complex, it requires someone competent in that field to explain and render an opinion. An expert witness doesn't necessarily have personal knowledge about the events. An expert witness can render testimony based upon a review of documents and through presentation of hypothetical facts.

Before an expert witness can testify at trial, the judge must determine that expert testimony is needed and that the expert has the necessary qualifications to render opinions. If the judge determines that the witness lacks the necessary qualifications, the judge may disqualify the expert witness and the expert will not be allowed to offer any opinion evidence.

Some States have established laws defining the qualifications necessary for a person to be qualified as an expert witness. Kansas requires that the testimony of expert witnesses must be in the form of opinions or inferences limited to such opinions as the judge finds are: (a) based on facts or data perceived by or personally known or made known to the expert witness at the trial; and (b) within the scope of the special knowledge, skill, experience, or training possessed by the expert witness.[4]

In *Tuck v. Health Care Authority of the City of Huntsville*[5], the judge refused to allow the expert witness to testify because she was not similarly situated as required by Alabama law. The case involved a hospitalized patient who was identified as being at risk for a fall so the fall-management protocol was initiated. The patient worked her way out of the restraint, got out of bed, and fell, breaking her hip. The primary issue was the standard of care in applying restraints.

The plaintiff's expert witness was a professor of sociology in nursing at Georgia State University with a Bachelor's of Science Degree of Nursing, a Master's of Science Degree in Medical-Surgery, and a Doctor of Philosophy Degree in Medical Sociology, Social Psychology Theory Development and Psychology. Despite this impressive credentials, she testified she had not been a staff nurse at a hospital since 1978 and she had last worked as a nurse in 1992. Since 1978, she had not taught clinical nursing courses, and had never used the type of belt restraint that was used on the patient. She further testified she had never written about patient restraints, she was not an expert on restraints, and she did not consider herself similarly situated to the nurses who had applied the restraints the patient.

The law in Alabama defines "similarly situated healthcare provider" as a person who: (a) is licensed by the appropriate regulatory board or agency; (b) is trained and experienced in the same discipline or school of practice; and (c) has

---

4   K.S.A. § 60-456(b).

5   851 S.2d 498 (Ala. 2002).

practiced in the same discipline or school of practice *during the year proceeding* the date that the alleged breach of the standard of care occurred.[6] The court determined that plaintiff's expert witness was *not* qualified to render opinions about the applicable standards of care. As a result of disqualify the expert witness, the Hospital's motion for judgment as a matter of law was granted and the lawsuit was dismissed.

The expert witness must define what the appropriate standards of care for the defendant nurse were *at the time* and *under the circumstances* of the alleged act. These may be based upon documents such as accreditation standards, practice standards, authoritative texts, journal articles, State or Federal laws, internal standards of the facility, or clinical practice guidelines, or just the expert's knowledge and experience.

An expert witness must also testify *what specific acts* constituted deviations from the standards of care. The testimony must be that these acts were deviations to a reasonable degree of nursing certainty. The expert's opinion must be more than a mere possibility or personal belief. It must be substantiated to prove that it is based on recognized standards of care and that the nurse's actions or omissions constituted deviations from those standards of care.

SECTION 4-5: TRIAL TESTIMONY

Testifying at trial is substantially different than testifying in a deposition. Prior to the trial, visit the courtroom and become familiar with its layout. Just knowing how to get to the courthouse, where to park, where the courtroom is, and where you are to sit can significantly alleviate some of the initial anxiety.

Spend time reviewing all pertinent documents and records and discuss the subject matter of the testimony in depth with the attorney requesting your appearance. The attorney should highlight anticipated areas of cross-examination so they can be discussed and thought given as to how those questions can be best answered.

Testifying at trial may be either by agreement or in response to a subpoena. A subpoena compels a witness to be present. If a subpoena is received, contact the attorney issuing the subpoena to determine exactly when your testimony is needed. Most attorneys will attempt to work with a witness in arranging a time that is convenient with the witness's schedule.

An important aspect of a witness's testimony is the witness's appearance and demeanor. How the witness dresses will create the jury's first impression of the witness. By sitting up and forward in the witness chair, this implies interest and confidence of the witness. Direct answers toward the jury as eye contact with

---

6 § 6-5-548, Alabama Code.

jurors is of extreme importance. They determine the credibility of witnesses which is a crucial factor when rendering a verdict. The jury must believe that the witness is interested, sincere, and confident about facts and opinions rendered.

Jurors have a great deal of respect for nurses and are reluctant to find fault with them. They see nursing as a benevolent profession. Most have been patients and been cared for by nurses so they know treatment is dependent on the existence of an intimate personal relationship between the nurse and patient. This relationship is further built on trust and confidence. That trusting relationship also invokes a willingness to forgive mistakes or accept unfortunate results. However, if the jurors perceive that the trust has been violated, they will react with a strong empathic sense of betrayal that results in moral outrage and indignation. Work to maintain that trust.

Recognize that the role of the opposing attorney is to discredit, confuse, point out ambiguities and differences in opinions, and destroy confidence. This is not a personal attack but is for the benefit of the jury and that attorney's client. However, if the jury believes the attorney is being unfair or demeaning to the witness, the jury tends to empathize and side with the witness. Avoid escalating any heated questioning. Respond calmly, and it will be the attorney who angers the jury.

At all times be respectful, courteous, and considerate with all individuals present in the courtroom. This includes the judge, attorneys, court reporter, bailiff, and jurors, as well as other witnesses and parties. Always be punctual for trial appearances. Understand courtroom etiquette, such as rising when the judge or jury enters and leaves the courtroom, witness procedures, and how to address the judge. This also creates a favorable impression upon the jury.

Even when not testifying or when court is not in session, the jury is constantly watching the attorneys and witnesses. Therefore, conduct must be closely controlled when anywhere near the courthouse.

At trial, witnesses are usually examined by both plaintiff and defendant attorneys. Frequently the attorney initially asking a witness questions at trial is eliciting favorable testimony, referred to as direct examination. In this format, the attorney asks very broad, open-ended questions to which more extensive and narrative answers are given. Trial *is* the time to teach and be helpful so that adequate explanations and information are provided to the jury.

Teach the jury those important facets and issues of the case, such as anatomy and physiology, the disease, standards of care, and alternative explanations for a patient's outcome. Talk to the jury as if teaching patients and clients. Avoid using technical terms and provide detailed explanations about the subject at issue. Prior to testifying, assist the attorney in developing appropriate visual aids that can be beneficial during trial, such as anatomy charts, diagrams, and enlarged medical records. Practice with them to make certain that the jury's view will not be blocked when using visual aids and that they can be seen and read by all jurors.

After direct examination is concluded, the adversarial attorney then cross-examines the witness. Cross-examination at trial usually is in the format of the attorney making a statement and asking the witness to agree with that statement, attempting to limit the witness to answer only "yes" or "no." To the extent possible, provide answers in your own words rather than merely allowing the attorney to testify for you. But remember that answers can be further explained later in redirect examination.

The other guidelines applicable in depositions are equally applicable in trial. Be adequately prepared, and have a sincere commitment to be an effective witness.

SECTION 4-6: DAMAGES

Damages awarded in a trial are either compensatory or punitive. Compensatory damages are intended to fully compensate the plaintiff to the extent possible for physical, financial, and emotional injuries. They compensate the concrete losses that the plaintiff has suffered because of defendant's wrongful conduct. Punitive damages have long been available to punish reprehensible conduct and to deter others from engaging in similar conduct. They are properly imposed to further a State's legitimate interests in punishing unlawful conduct. Thus, compensatory and punitive damages are awarded at the same time by the same decision maker but for different purposes.

Excessive punitive damage awards are of special concern in today's cost-conscious healthcare environment. Anxiety is high about the willingness of juries to award millions and even billions of dollars in punitive damages.

Although States possess discretion over how punitive damages can be imposed, the basis for them and the amount, there are procedural and substantive constitutional limitations on these awards. Repeatedly the United States Supreme Court has been asked to address issues related to punitive damages from the perspective of whether they violate the due process clause of the Fourteenth Amendment because they are grossly excessive or arbitrary punishments. As the Supreme Court has noted: "To the extent an award is grossly excessive, it furthers no legitimate purpose and constitutes an arbitrary deprivation of property."[7] The Supreme Court has also noted that punitive damage awards serve the same purposes as criminal penalties and yet defendants are subjective to punitive damages without having the same protections applicable in criminal proceedings.[8]

---

7 *Pacific Mutual Life Insurance Company v. Haslip*, 499 U.S. 1, 111 S.Ct. 1032, 113 L.Ed.2d 1 (1991).

8 *State Farm Mutual Automobile Insurance Company v. Campbell*, 123 S.Ct. 1513, 1520, 155 L.Ed.2d 585 (2003).

Prior to 1996, the Supreme Court was hesitant to impose a Federal check on the amount of punitive damages awarded in State courts. In 1996, for the first time the Supreme Court validated a punitive damages assessment as unreasonably large.[9] In that case, three guideposts were established for reviewing punitive damages: (1) the degree of reprehensibility of the defendant's misconduct; (2) the disparity between the actual or potential harm suffered by the plaintiff and the punitive damages award; and (3) the difference between the punitive damages awarded by the jury and the penalties authorized or imposed in comparable cases.[10]

In *Campbell,* the Supreme Court used those three criteria to evaluate the award of $145 million in punitive damages when only $1 million in compensatory damages had been awarded. As the Supreme Court noted, "It should be presumed the plaintiff has been made whole for injuries sustained by compensatory damages, the punitive damages should only be awarded if the defendant's culpability, after having paid compensatory damages, is so reprehensible as to warrant the imposition of further sanctions to achieve punishment or deterrence.[11]

The reasonableness of a punitive damages award must reflect the reprehensibility of the defendant's conduct. To determine the reprehensibility of a defendant, the following must be determined: (1) whether the harm caused was physical as opposed to economic; (2) was the tortuous conduct evidence of indifference to or a reckless disregard of the health or safety of others; (3) did the target of the conduct have financial vulnerability; (4) did the conduct involve repeated actions or was an isolated incident; and (5) did the harm result from intentional malice, trickery, deceit, or mere accident.[12]

Historically, the Supreme Court rejected the notation that a simple mathematical formula could establish the constitutional line between compensatory and punitive damages. Over the past 700 years, sanctions of double, triple, or quadruple damages have typically been awarded to deter and punish. "All of these ratios are not binding, they are instructive."[13]

In analyzing the award of $145 million in punitive damages, the Supreme Court noted that the compensatory damages of $1 million was substantial for the year and a half of emotional distress sustained by the Campbells. Must of the distress was caused by the outrage and humiliation the Campbells suffered as a result of the actions of State Farm. In its reasoning, the Supreme Court decided: "The punitive award of $145 million, therefore, was neither reasonable nor pro-

---

9 *BMW of North America, Inc. v. Gore,* 517 U.S. 559, 116 S.Ct. 1589 134 L.Ed.2d 809 (1996).

10 *Id.* at 575.

11 *Campbell, supra* at 1521.

12 *Id.* at 1521.

13 *Id.* at 1524.

portionate to the wrong committed, and it was an irrational and arbitrary deprivation of the property of the defendant."[14]

This recent decision by the U.S. Supreme Court will be the guiding case law for future punitive damage awards.

SECTION 4-7: CASE STUDIES

A. Personal Injury

Mary Jones was 83 years of age when she suffered a stroke. She was placed in a long-term care facility, Nursing Homes, Inc. As a result of the stroke, Mrs. Jones is virtually paralyzed from the neck down. In addition, for a few months she could not speak.

When Mrs. Jones was admitted to Nursing Homes, Inc., her daughter discussed with the staff the care required to prevent decubitus ulcers. However, within a week of admission to Nursing Homes, Inc., Mrs. Jones developed decubitus ulcers on her shoulder and upper back. Fortunately, they quickly healed.

In January, Mrs. Jones developed pneumonia. At this time, her daughter requested that she be placed on a no-code status. However, Mrs. Jones subsequently rallied and overcame the pneumonia.

Beginning in January, Mrs. Jones developed decubitus ulcers on her heels, in particular her right heel. She also developed a decubitus ulcer on the back of her left thigh. Mrs. Jones' daughter believes that Duoderm patches placed on her mother's decubitus ulcers were changed on an irregular basis. She alleges that there was no consistency in following the doctor's orders as to changing the Duoderm patches. In April, Mrs. Jones was taken to a hospital for surgical debridement of her left heel.

While Mrs. Jones was at Nursing Homes, Inc., she also developed a "horrible mouth fungus." Her physician told her daughter that the fungus was caused by oral hygiene neglect. He stated that there was evidence she had retained flood in her mouth which had not been properly cleaned out between meals.

Mrs. Jones' daughter alleges that she was told by several members of the nursing staff that the Administrator was totally incompetent as an administrative person and had no idea how work should be done at a long-terms care facility. Those same employees also allegedly told Mrs. Jones' daughter that Nursing Homes, Inc., was too cheap to hire proper personnel and thus the care was inadequate. The daughter also identified three employees whom she though provided inadequate care and described them as being "pitifully incompetent, hopelessly dull, hateful, and extremely lazy."

---

14 *Id.* at 1526.

On several occasions, Mrs. Jones' daughter had meetings with the Administrator and Director of Nursing regarding their complaints about their mother's care. They also had numerous complaints about the condition of the nursing home. They stated that the facility was often dirty and unhealthy. Several instances were cited when the washing machine was not functioning and thus there were not enough clean linens available. On several occasions, there was no laundry soap and linens had been washed anyway. Instances were when her mother received the wrong dietary tray at mealtime. Mrs. Jones was on a puree diet but received a regular diet tray and thus could not swallow the food.

Mrs. Jones' daughter began writing a diary concerning her mother's condition because she believed that she was not receiving proper care. This diary contained references to a variety of complaints. Finally, in May, Mrs. Jones' daughter filed a complaint with the Division of Aging. An investigator came to the facility and met with Mrs. Jones' daughter. There was subsequent citations issued against the nursing home based upon the care of Mrs. Jones.

B. Wrongful Death

Patient Risky was brought to the Emergency Department at Quality Hospital at approximately 4:30 p.m.. She was a 44 year old woman with Down's Syndrome who had choked on a piece of beef stew at supper that evening. Mrs. Risky had a past history of ingesting foreign bodies, including a glass light bulb. Based on her symptoms, the Emergency Department physician called in a general surgeon and ENT specialist.

At approximately 7:35 p.m., the physicians performed a laryngoscopy and rigid esophagoscopy with removal of a foreign body. The procedure was completed at approximately 8 p.m. The patient was kept in the recovery room until she was taken to the medical/surgical floor at approximately 10 p.m. However, no records from the recovery room have been located.

Susie Careless, RN came on duty at 11 p.m. She normally worked in labor and delivery but was floated to the medical/surgical floor because of lack of staffing. Although her shift was scheduled to end at 7 a.m. on March 24, she was told that she had to work another shift due to lack of staffing.

Nurse Careless admits that at the time of the incident in question she was not aware of the potential complications after an esophagoscopy. Since then, she has done extensive reading and is now knowledgeable regarding them.

Nurse Careless alleges she checked on Patient Risky more frequently than documented. She would not document if the condition was essentially the same.

Nurse Careless is aware that normal respirations are between 16 and 22. She was aware that the patient's respirations were elevated and there was some distress noted. She attributed this to increased anxiety and activity. She did not believe they were significant enough to notify Dr. Smith.

Nurse Careless acknowledged that Patient Risky made frequent complaints about lower back pain and a sore throat. At the time she did not realize that those were symptoms of a perforated esophagus. She encouraged fluids to provide relief.

Nurse Careless is aware that it is important to evaluate respiratory functioning in any patient but even more so in a patient post-laryngoscopy and esophagoscopy. This evaluation should include assessment of lung sounds, the patient's appearance, and pattern of breath sounds. Nurse Careless is aware that shallow breathing, retractions, and a patient's color may be indicators of respiratory distress. She did note these on several occasions.

Nurse Careless testifies that when Dr. Smith made rounds at 9 a.m., she advised him about the patient's condition. However, that conversation was not documented and Nurse Careless cannot recall exactly what she told Dr. Smith. She is aware that Dr. Smith does not routinely read nurses' notes.

Nurse Careless does not believe the elevated temperature was of any significance in Patient Risky. She attributed this to a normal reaction post-esophagoscopy. Therefore, she would not have particularly brought that to Dr. Smith's attention.

Although Nurse Careless charted "Fleets enema given" at 1 p.m., she testifies that was given by a nursing assistant. She does not remember who that was. Nurse Careless did not observe the patient during the enema nor observe the results. These were also reported by the nursing assistant.

Nurse Careless admitted that she was notified by Patient Risky's sister at 2:25 p.m. that the patient was in distress. At that time, she found the patient cyanotic and having labored respirations. However, because she had neglected to call the nursing supervisor to restart the IV which had been pulled out at 1:30 p.m., she first contacted the supervisor so that the IV could be restarted prior to calling the physician. She then notified the physician at 3 p.m.

Nurse Careless acknowledged that the physician had ordered vital signs to be taken very one hour x 3; then every four hours. She stated that she was unable to take vital signs as frequently as ordered because she had too many patients to care for. She also cannot account for the discrepancy between the vital signs documented on the graphic record and in the nurses' records for 10 p.m.

REFERENCES

Birholz, G., *Malpractice Data from the National Practitioner Data Bank*, 20 The Nurse Practitioner 32 (March 1995).

Fiesta, J., *Communication—The Value of An Apology*, 25 Nursing Management 14 (August 1994).

Filkins, James A., *With No Evil Intent*, 22 The Journal of Legal Medicine 467 (2001).

Fink, S. and Chaudhuri, T. K., *Medical Characteristics of 61 Unwarranted Malpractice Claims*, 88 Southern Medical Journal 1011 (October 1995).

Geertsma, Meleah A., *Recent Developments in Health Law: Punitive Damages*, 31 J. of Law, Medicine and Ethics 308 (Summer 2003).

Infante, Marie C., *Malpractice May Not Be Your Biggest Legal Risk*, 63 RN 67 (July 2000).

Kohn, L. T., Corrigan, J. M., and Donaldson, M. S., (editors), Institute of Medicine, Chapter 6: *Protecting Voluntary Reporting Systems From Legal Discovery*, To Err Is Human: Building A Safer Health System. (2000).

Ladebauche, P., *Limiting Liability to Avoid Malpractice Litigation*, 20 MCN 243 (September/October 1995).

Miller-Slade, Donna, *Liability Theories In Nursing Negligence Cases*, 52 Trial (May 1997).

Murray, Marilyn Kettering, *The Nursing Shortage: Past, Present and Future*, 32 JONA 79 (February 2002).

Purnell, L., *What To Do If Called Upon To Testify*, 3 Accid Emergency Nurs 19 (January 1995).

Sarhaddi, Richard C., *Peer Review Immunity And The Health Care Quality Improvement Act*, 7 CCH Healthcare Compliance Letter (October 27, 2003).

Saxton, James W., *Making Risk Management Positive and Mandatory*, 6 Healthcare Liability and Litigation (2003).

Shaw, Robert Ward, *Punitive Damages In Medical Malpractice: An Economical Evaluation*, 81 North Carolina Law Rev. 2371 (2003).

Solon, M., *Nurses and the Law: A Growing Band of Expert Witnesses*, 9 Nursing Standards 21 (January 1995).

Tokarski, Cathy, *Malpractice Reform Signed Into Law in Florida*, Medscape Medical News (2003), at http://www.medscape.com/viewarticle/461009.

United States Chamber of Commerce, U.S. Chamber of Commerce State Liability Systems Ranking Study (January 11, 2002).

Wright, J. Kim and Garlo, Dolly M. *Visionary Law: New Approaches Expand Choices In Law Practice*, 8 Journal of Nursing Law 7 (2002).

CHAPTER 5

Professional Licensure: Regulatory Issues and Legal Actions

SECTION 5-1: NURSING REGULATORY AGENCIES AND NURSE PRACTICE ACTS

"Lax government oversight and a shoddy system of reporting medical errors allows negligent, incompetent and impaired registered nurses to return to work in Illinois even after committing deadly errors . . . registered nurses have injected themselves with heroine and cocaine, then committed dozens of errors. . . . [Nurses] have been convicted of felony crimes, from child molesting to drug trafficking and have killed."[1] These are the statements read by the public, and certainly such statements aren't limited to this one article. Nursing regulatory agencies have been criticized for patterns of leniency toward problem nurses and lacking resources to identify those nurses posing potential dangers.

Through mandated licensing of professional nurses, the public's health, safety, and welfare are protected from potential harm by those who lack the necessary competency to practice. All States require licensure for individuals who wish to practice nursing. Through legislation, standards are set for entry into practice, the scope of nursing practice is defined; and a State nursing regulatory agency is established to implement licensing functions, enact regulations, and adjudicate disciplinary actions.

The Governor of the State generally appoints the members of the State nursing regulatory agency. Laws designate the number of members, usually from

---

1 Berens, M. J., *Problem Nurses Escape Punishment*, Chicago Tribune (September 12, 2000).

three to twenty (although the majority have no more than ten) and the composition of the members, which usually includes representation from various areas or specialties in nursing and with members having a minimum number of years in nursing practice. The nursing regulatory agency is presumed to be qualified to exercise its authority and to make decisions based upon appropriate standards.

The nursing regulatory agency may be accused of abusing its authority and discretion when taking action against a nurse's license. This was the issue in *Burns v. Board of Nursing of Iowa.*[2] The Iowa Board of Nursing found Joann Burns habitually intoxicated and placed her nursing license on probation for three years, with several stringent conditions. Nurse Burns challenged the Board's action, alleging that it was not supported by substantial evidence and that the Board abused its discretion by imposing stringent conditions upon her.

Nurse Burns became a registered nurse on December 1, 1960. From September 9, 1968, she was continuously employed by a Mason City hospital. There were indications that Nurse Burns misused alcohol on November 5, 1986, June 20, 1989, and January 18, 1990. Regarding the November 5th incident, the supervisor for Nurse Burns confronted her regarding the odor of alcohol that was noted by ancillary personnel. Nurse Burns advised that it would not happen again. The supervisor issued an oral warning.

Subsequently, the hospital became convinced that Nurse Burns had a serious problem with alcohol. Two other nurses smelled alcohol on Nurse Burns while she was on duty. One nurse stated this happened as often as once every two weeks. Nurse Burns was sometimes seen eating lemon which was interpreted as evidence of hiding the alcohol's distinctive odor.

She was increasingly absent and was compelled to withdraw from chemotherapy training "due to tremulous hands."

Following another confrontation between Nurse Burns and her supervisor because of the odor of alcohol on Nurse Burns, Nurse Burns was demoted from her position as charge nurse. She was required to be assessed by the hospital's alcohol and drug recovery program. Evidently when Nurse Burns called the program director for an appointment, her slurred words and inappropriate comments convinced the program director that Nurse Burns was intoxicated at the time. Testifying as an expert, the program director stated that common symptoms of alcohol abuse in nurses include denial, physical changes, and general changes in behavior, including job performance. She also stated that nurses generally abuse alcohol for a minimum of three to five years prior to the time it is detected in the work place. The problem is finally detected at work, by absenteeism, failure to perform some quantity or quality of work as previously performed, and the tendency to avoid challenging assignments.

2 528 N.W.2d 602 (Iowa 1995).

In June 1990, the Iowa Board of Nursing found Nurse Burns was habitually intoxicated as charged and placed her nursing license on probation. It further required Nurse Burns to receive inpatient treatment for her alcohol problem followed by after care treatment, attend Alcoholics Anonymous, submit to random blood or urine testing, and undergo a medical and psychiatric examination at her own expense within three months of the end of the probation. Nurse Burns sought judicial review of the Board's action.

Nurse Burns actually sought judicial review in two separate proceedings. In *Burns v. Board of Nursing*,[3] she challenged whether the finding of habitual intoxication was supported by substantial evidence. The court agreed with the Board's view that it must be allowed to determine whether a nurse is habitually intoxicated on a case by case basis in light of public health and safety concerns. A specific definition of what constitutes "habitual intoxication" would be inadequate for the Board's purposes in overseeing the licensing of nurses. As the court noted: "The nursing board is called upon to defend the public interest in the crucial and exacting matter of health care. In doing so, it cannot be held to the showing of habitual intoxication required for such things as involuntary treatment."[4]

The court emphasized that the Board was not required to wait to take action until the habitual intoxication becomes so debilitating that there is immediate danger of harm to patients. The Board's mandate is to protect the public by taking action when harm is imminent or before it occurs. The court concluded that Nurse Burns was habitually intoxicated when her repeated ingestion of alcohol compromised her professional capacity while on duty and therefore threatened the safety of hospital patients subject to her care.[5]

In her second appeal, Nurse Burns questioned the stringent terms of probation as being unreasonable and beyond the Board's authority. In examining the terms of probation imposed by the Board, the court discussed the Board's authority:

> A professional licensing board's authority to impose sanctions against those it licenses is extremely broad. The purpose of statutory licensing schemes is to protect the public health, safety and welfare of the people of Iowa. We therefore construe licensing statutes liberally to carry out that purpose. (Citations omitted.)[6]

---

3 495 N.W.2d 698 (Iowa 1993).

4 *Id.* at 700–701.

5 *Id.* at 701.

6 *Burns, supra*, at 604.

The court interpreted "an abuse of discretion" as being synonymous with unreasonableness. It defined unreasonableness as "action in the face of evidence as to which there is no room for a difference of opinion among reasonable minds or not based on substantial evidence."[7] The court upheld the Board's terms of probation by noting: "When the licensing Board is made up of members of the profession they are licensing, the court should not second guess the Board's discretion to determine what conditions should be attached to probation."[8]

In 1996, the National Council of State Boards of Nursing issued a paper addressing the regulation of nursing.[9] The conclusion were:

- Regulation implies the intervention of the government to accomplish an end beneficial to its citizens

- The Tenth Amendment reserves to the States all powers not delegated to the United Stated by the US Constitution.

- The power to regulate occupations as based upon the power of the State to enact reasonable laws necessary to protect its citizens.

- Regulatory authority is derived from legislative action.

- State legislatures delegate many enforcement activities to State administrative agencies.

- The delegation of regulatory authority allows the legislature to use the expertise of the agencies and the implementation of statutes.

While recognizing the benefits of regulation, the National Council recognized the current challenges, especially as a barrier to health care access. Thus began exploring whether some licensure activities could be centralized while still maintaining the protections of state authority for nursing practice.

In July 1999, the National Council of State Boards of Nursing issued its position on "Uniform Core Licensure Requirements."[10] The paper was the result of the National Council's Nursing Practice and Education Committee working for two years to develop core licensure requirements. The premises of the committee are:

---

7 *Id.* at 605.

8 *Id.* at 605.

9 National Council of State Boards of Nursing, *Public Protection of Professional Self-Preservation? The Purpose of Regulation*, The National Council Staff Presentation (1996), at http://www.ncsbn.org/.

10 *National Council of State Boards of Nursing, Uniform Core Licensure Requirements: A Supporting Paper*, National Council of State Boards of Nursing (July 1999).

- It is critical to focus on what the public needs rather than what States are currently doing.

- It is desirable to divide the huge challenge of Uniform Licensure requirements into manageable sections.

- It is crucial to avoid simply choosing the least common denominator.

- It is important to avoid redundancy in the requirements.

- It is important to define "core" to mean minimum and essential.

- It is essential that member boards continue to be responsible for verification that nurses meet these uniform requirements.

- It is assumed that boards that approve the uniform core licensure requirements will have a reasonable approach to verifying these requirements.

- The underlying goal is to promote public safety in the least restrictive manner.

To achieve uniform core licensure requirements requires: willingness to place emphasis on the public good; willingness to compromise; and willingness to trust sister nurse regulatory agencies.

To date, a number of States have adopted the Nurse Licensure Compact:

State	Implementation Date
Arizona	July 2002
Arkansas	July 2000
Delaware	July 2000
Idaho	July 2001
Indiana	To Be Determined
Iowa	July 2000
Maine	July 2001
Maryland	July 1999
Mississippi	July 2001
Nebraska	January 2001
New Jersey	To Be Determined
New Mexico	July 2004
North Carolina	July 2000
North Dakota	January 2004

South Dakota	January 2001
Tennessee	July 2003
Texas	January 2000
Utah	January 2000
Virginia	January 2005
Wisconsin	January 2000[11]

Unlike licensure requirements for RNs and LPN/LVNs (which are generally similar among the States) requirements and approaches for regulating advanced practice registered nurses is quite varied from State to State and among APRN categories within the State. The National Council of State Boards of Nursing (NCSBN) designated an APRN Task Force to develop uniform requirements for mutual recognition of APRNs across States. The Uniform APRN model language was approved by the NCSBN Delegate Assembly on August 16, 2002. A State must either have adopted the *Nurse Licensure Compact* for RNs and LPNs, adopt both Compacts simultaneously to be eligible for the APRN Compact.[12]

SECTION 5-2: COMPLAINTS: INVESTIGATION; PROCEDURES; DUE PROCESS

A. Initiation of Investigation

Nursing regulatory agencies are required to investigate complaints filed against nurses, and to discipline nurses who violate the laws of the State. Malpractice claims involving nurses that are settled or result in judgments awarded must be reported to State nursing regulatory agencies under the Health Care Quality Improvement Act (HCQIA). Many States mandate that reports be made regarding nurses who have violated the State Nurse Practice Act, are impaired due to drugs or alcohol, or against whom disciplinary action has been taken by an employer. Patients are more frequently submitting complaints about nurses. All of these must be thoroughly investigated to meet statutory duties to the public.

State laws define the requirements for how a complaint is made. Typically it must be in writing, include the nurse's full name, and license number if known, describe the incident, and identify the person reporting the complaint.

---

11 *The Nurse Licensure Compact* as adopted and information about individual State Nurse Practice Acts can be accessed at http://www.ncsbn.org/.

12 The *APRN Compact* as adopted and information about individual State Nurse Practice Acts can be accessed at http://www.ncsbn.org/.

When received, a complaint is reviewed and a determination made whether more information is needed from the complainant, whether an investigation is needed, or whether it can be closed with no action being taken.

If the nursing regulatory agency requests information, read the request immediately, note the date the response is due, and contact an attorney.[13] It is imperative to have legal representation during the course of the investigation since anything said during the investigation can be used against the nurse in a subsequent hearing. Additionally, the information provided during the investigation is the determining factor as to whether disciplinary action will be taken against the nurse. Attorneys are in a much better position to adequately represent the nurse, make certain appropriate information is communicated to the investigator and regulatory agency, and to assist in appropriately resolving any issues.

The nurse's professional liability insurance policy may provide coverage for the legal fees and costs required to respond to the investigation. Contact the insurance company and request an attorney be provided for representation during the investigation.

If an investigator telephones requesting information or shows up unannounced, be cordial, but insist on speaking with your attorney prior to answering any questions. There is no legal obligation to immediately talk with the investigator or release any records, other than as set forth in a subpoena.

Prior to meeting with the investigator, meet with your attorney to discuss the issues and concerns that are being investigated. Have a copy of the complaint or an understanding of the basis for the investigation. Carefully review all health information related to the patient or incident. Conversations with other health care providers should occur only with an attorney present to protect the confidentiality of those communications. Otherwise, the people present during those meetings can be questioned about what was said, which can create the perception of attempting to cover up or change testimony that may be adverse to the nurse.

After meeting with the investigator, a written response to all of the allegations can be prepared and submitted to the regulatory agency for consideration along with the investigator's report. Include supporting literature and letters from other nurses and physicians.

If requested to meet with the regulatory agency, always appear with an attorney. Similarly, do not sign a stipulation or disciplinary agreement with the regulatory agency without the advice of legal counsel; it can't be reversed!

---

13 LaDuke, S., *Yes, You Need A Lawyer*, 31 Nursing 2001 61 (March 2001).

B. DUE PROCESS

If a disciplinary action against a nurse is pursued, the nurse is entitled to certain rights as defined by the State's administrative procedure act or other State laws. Know what these rights are because the failure to exercise them timely *will* result in their waiver!

These rights guarantee nurses due process. The Due Process Clause of the U.S. Constitution prevents a person from being deprived of life, liberty, or property. Founded upon fundamental principles of justice; it ensures the fair and orderly administration of laws and protects nurses from arbitrary actions.

The two primary elements of due process are that: (1) the rules as applied must be reasonable and definite; and (2) fair procedures must be followed in enforcing the rules. These elements require that nurses have knowledge that the questioned conduct is prohibited (sometimes referred to as "adequate notice"). Frequent challenges to regulatory agency result because of alleged "vagueness of the law."

The test for determining unconstitutional vagueness is whether the language of the regulation is so vague, with respect to what conduct is either proscribed or required, that persons of common intelligence must necessarily guess at its meaning. The words can't invite arbitrary decision-making.

The other element of due process provides the nurse with: (1) adequate notice of the time and place of the hearing; (2) the right to be represented by an attorney at the hearing; (3) the right to subpoena witnesses on the nurse's behalf and present evidence at the hearing; (4) the right to cross-examine witnesses; (5) the right to a record of the proceeding; and (6) the right to a review of the regulatory agency's decision by a court.

To adequately prepare for a hearing, discovery proceeds in the same manner and on the same conditions as provided for in other legal proceedings.

In legal actions parties are entitled to obtain discovery regarding any matter not privileged which is relative to the subject matter involved in the pending action. The rules of discovery are liberally construed.

C. Hearings

The form of the disciplinary hearing varies among States. It may be conducted by the nurse regulatory agency or by administrative judges. The evidentiary rules are not strictly adhered to in the hearing so evidence is admitted that would not otherwise be admitted in a trial court. Expert witnesses are frequently used. The decision must be based *only* on the evidence presented at the hearing. The amount of proof is usually substantial evidence—evidence that is persuasive and adequate to support a conclusion.

Actions that may be taken against nurses are set forth in State laws. These may include: reprimand; probation; suspension; the placing of specific conditions on the licensee such as requiring supervision; forbidding involvement in certain activities like prescribing or administering medications; requiring additional education; or revocation. If a disciplinary action against a nurse results from substance abuse, the nurse may be referred to an impaired nurse program if the State has such a program recognized by the regulatory agency. With an impaired nurse, the focus is rehabilitation. Provided that the nurse successfully completes the rehabilitation program, the regulatory agency may choose to not pursue any disciplinary action.

SECTION 5-3: GROUNDS FOR DISCIPLINE

Each State defines what grounds may result in disciplinary action by the nursing regulatory agency. Possible violations for which disciplinary actions may be instigated include:

1. Conviction of a felony or crime involving moral turpitude;
2. Use of fraud or deceit in obtaining licensure;
3. Violation of the provisions of the nurse practice act;
4. Aiding or abetting any unlicensed person with the unauthorized practice of nursing;
5. Revocation, suspension, or denial of licensure to practice nursing in any other state;
6. Habitual use of, or addiction to, alcohol or drugs;
7. Unprofessional conduct; and
8. Lack of fitness by reason of physical or mental health that could result in injury to the public.

A. Unprofessional Conduct

Because under due process the nurse must be afforded adequate notice of what conduct is prohibited by law, frequently appeals are based upon the lack of clarity in defining misconduct, especially regarding what constitutes "unprofessional conduct."

Whether a nurse's actions constituted "unprofessional conduct" was addressed by the court in *Stephens v. Pennsylvania State Board of Nursing.*[14] Paula Stephens, L.P.N., was found by the Pennsylvania State Board of Nursing to have engaged in unprofessional conduct, for which the Board formally repri-

---

14 657 A.2d 71 (Pa. Cmwlth. 1995).

manded Nurse Stephens and assessed a civil penalty in the amount of $1,000. The grounds for the Board's decision are the following findings of fact:

1. From April 1985 until October 1989, Nurse Stephens was employed as a charge nurse at State College Manor Nursing Home with some supervisory authority over several nurse aides.

2. In late summer or early fall 1988, Timothy Berrena, a nurse aide at State College Manor Nursing Home, in the presence of Nurse Stephens, ingested a small amount of Haldol which Nurse Stephens had poured for a patient.

3. In August 1988, Nurse Aide Berrena, in the presence of Nurse Stephens, verbally and physically harassed an elderly infirm resident by flicking the resident's hat and otherwise verbally teasing the resident and causing him to become increasingly agitated.

4. Nurse Stephens allowed Nurse Aide Berrena's harassment of the resident to continue for approximately ten minutes before taking action to stop it.

5. Nurse Stephens did not report either the incident involving Nurse Aide Berrena ingesting resident medication nor Nurse Aide Berrena's harassment of a resident to a supervising nurse or to any other person of authority at the nursing home.

The Board concluded: Nurse Stephens' failure to report Nurse Aide Berrena after he ingested the medication prescribed for a resident constituted unprofessional conduct; Nurse Stephens' observation of Nurse Aide Berrena's harassment of the resident for approximately ten minutes before she took action to stop it constituted unprofessional conduct; and Nurse Stephens' failure to report Nurse Aide Berrena after he harassed the resident constituted unprofessional conduct.

A vague statute denies due process by "(1) not giving fair notice to people of ordinary intelligence that their contemplated activity may be unlawful and (2) they do not set reasonably clear guidelines for law officials and courts, thus inviting arbitrary and discriminatory enforcement."[15] But the court further noted that this language may be interpreted in the context of the common knowledge and understanding of members of a particular profession to determine if it gains the required specificity.

As the Board wrote in its decision, "It is incumbent upon a nurse to look out for the welfare of all patients." Nurse Stephens' failure to report Nurse Aide Berrena for either instance was evidence of poor judgment and deplorable

---

15 *Id.* at 74.

behavior that rises to the level of unprofessional conduct. The term gains the required specificity when considered within the context of the common knowledge and practices of members of the practical nursing profession. What standard of conduct is expected of a licensed practical nurse is defined in Pennsylvania: "licensed practical nurse shall, inter alia, respect a patient's right to freedom from physical abuse and act to safeguard a patient from abusive practice of any individual. Further, a licensed practical nurse may not knowingly assist another person to violate or circumvent a law or board regulation."[16]

The court concluded that Nurse Stephens was aware of what constituted unprofessional conduct and there was an ascertainable standard against which her conduct could be measured. The formal reprimanding and penalty of $1,000 assessed by the Board was upheld by the court.

In *Husher v. Commissioner of Education of the State of New York,*[17] Darlene Husher, both a registered nurse and licensed practical nurse, was charged with professional misconduct for abandoning her professional employment with the hospital and practicing nursing with gross negligence. Nurse Husher left her assigned nursing unit at a hospital without informing the staff remaining on the unit that she was leaving.

Nurse Husher was advised by her supervisor that, due to a staff shortage on the 3:00 p.m. to 11:00 p.m. shift, one of the 7:00 a.m. to 3:00 p.m. shift nurses would have to remain on duty. Under the hospital's mandatory overtime policy, the nurse with the least seniority was required to stay. Nurse Husher informed the supervisor that she would stay for several hours until properly relieved. Nurse Husher informed the staff on the unit that she was going to the supervisor's office and could be paged if an emergency arose. After conversing with the supervisor, Nurse Husher then left the hospital altogether without first returning to the unit to advise the staff that she was leaving and would not be available to respond in the event of an emergency. This left twenty-nine patients, most of whom were elderly and suffering from multiple illnesses, some were receiving intravenous therapy, and three who were intubated and on respirators unattended by a registered nurse and staffed only by nurses' aides, orderlies, and a respiratory therapist.

To support a finding of misconduct under New York law, there must be:

1. Abandonment of professional employment;
2. Without reasonable notice; and
3. Under circumstances which seriously impair the delivery of professional care to patients.

---

16 *Id.* at 75.

17 591 N.Y.S.2d 99 (N.Y. A.D. 1992).

The court upheld the findings of the hearing panel: (1) that the hospital had a bona fide overtime policy of which Nurse Husher was aware; (2) that as the nurse with least seniority she was required to remain on duty during an emergency situation; (3) that such an emergency situation existed because of a shortage of staff; (4) that Nurse Husher was aware of the emergency and she was advised by her supervisor that she would have to stay; (5) that she subsequently refused to do so; and (6) that she left the unit unattended by a registered nurse. Based upon these findings, the court agreed that Nurse Husher was guilty of professional misconduct and her licenses to practice as a registered nurse and licensed practice nurse would be suspended for one year.

Nurse Jose N. Proenza Sanfiel appealed an order issued by the Florida State Board of Nursing suspending his psychiatric nursing license and placing him on probation.[18] Proenza Sanfiel obtained a computer which was previously owned by Charter Behavioral Health System which still contained patient records. Nurse Proenza Sanfiel then called the news media and allowed them to see the patient information. He told the reporters that the computer contained the names of psychiatric patients, their admission dates, types of addiction, treatments, and psychiatric disorders. The media broadcasted this story along with the patient name and diagnoses. An unknown number of patients were contacted by the news reporters.

Nurse Proenza Sanfiel's nursing license was immediately suspended during the investigation. Nurse Proenza Sanfiel never disputed that he made the disclosure or that he was unaware that the information was confidential. His arguments were that the conduct did not involve patients under his care, and he was acting in a private capacity and not as a nurse to the patients. The law for which Nurse Proenza Sanfiel was disciplined was "Violating the confidentiality of information or knowledge concerning a patient." Grounds for the disciplinary action were "Knowingly violating any provisions of this chapter, a rule of the board or department, or a lawful order of the board or department previously entered in a disciplinary proceeding or failing to comply with a lawfully issued subpoena of the department."[19] Only if the interpretation of a statute or regulation by a regulatory agency should be given difference and not be overturned unless it is clearly erroneous. "So long as the agency's interpretation is within the range of possible and reasonable, it should be affirmed."[20] The court concluded that the board reasonably interpreted "unprofessional conduct" to include violating the confidentiality of information or knowledge concerning a patient.

---

18 *Proenza Sanfiel, RN v. Department of Health*, 749 So.2d 525 (Fla.App. 1999).

19 *Id.* at 526–527.

20 *Id.* at 527.

B. Willful Conduct

Courts frequently address whether failing to renew a nursing license constitutes willful conduct. Most have held that to prove this amounted to willful conduct, there must be evidence that the nurses were consciously aware that they were practicing without a license or that they willfully or intentionally failed to renew the license.

The North Dakota Supreme Court addressed this issue in *Sande v. State of North Dakota and the Board of Nursing of the State of North Dakota.*[21] Nancy Sande became a registered nurse in 1969. She renewed her license to practice nursing each year prior to 1987. During 1987, except for the month of May, Nurse Sande worked as a registered nurse. On the evening of November 12, 1987, Nurse Sande became aware that she did not have a 1987 license. She testified that she thought there was something wrong because she had not received a renewal form. The next day Nurse Sande went to the office of the Board of Nursing, met with the Executive Director, and renewed her license for 1987. She paid a late renewal fee of $40. The Executive Director told Nurse Sande she would be subject to an administrative proceeding for practicing nursing without a current license.

The Executive Director also submitted the information to the county's attorney. Nurse Sande was prosecuted for the misdemeanor offense of practicing as a registered nurse without being licensed. Nurse Sande agreed to a "Stipulation for Deferred Prosecution and Order" whereby Nurse Sande would not be required to enter a plea to the charge, prosecution would be deferred for six months, and the charge would be dismissed with prejudice if she did not violate any criminal laws during that time.

An administrative complaint was brought by the Board charging Nurse Sande for willful and repeated violations of practicing nursing without a license. At the hearing, the Executive Director testified that the Board mailed a license renewal form each October to every currently licensed nurse. There was no record that the form had been returned by the postal service as undelivered to Nurse Sande. Nurse Sande admitted that she was aware and conscious that a practicing nurse must have a current license, but testified that she did not realize that she was practicing in 1987 without a current license.

The Board concluded that during 1987: (1) Nurse Sande "willfully practiced as a registered nurse of her own free will and not under coercion;" (2) that Nurse Sande, "working a standard five day work week, did willfully and repeatedly practice as a registered nurse within North Dakota while she was not licensed by the Board as a registered nurse to perform those duties;" and (3) that it was Nurse Sande's "professional and legal duty to first seek and obtain such

21 440 N.W.2d 264 (N.D. 1989).

licensing prior to entering into her duties as a registered nurse." The Board assessed Nurse Sande a license penalty fee of $460 computed at $5 per day for 92 working days. The Board also directed that Nurse Sande be publicly reprimanded.

In its review, the court emphasized the finding of the Board must be affirmed: (1) if the findings of fact are supported by a preponderance of the evidence; (2) if the conclusions of law are sustained by the findings of fact; (3) if the Board decision is supported by the conclusions of law; and (4) if the decision is in accordance with the law.[22] The primary arguments centered upon the construction of "willfully" as used in the statute. The Board's contention was that the meaning of "willfully" should not be limited to acts performed with evil purpose, but should include any act voluntarily undertaken regardless of whether the nurse was conscious that the act constituted a violation. Nurse Sande argued that "willfully" should require proof that she was consciously aware of her violation of a statutory obligation.

The court took notice that the Board treated each day that Nurse Sande practiced without a current license as a separate violation to meet the repeat element that was required under the statute and disagreed with the Board's interpretation:

> A "repeated" violation is usually viewed as a failure to comply with a standard about which a person should be conscious because of prior citations or violations. The Legislature's requirement that a violation be not only "willful" but also "repeated" clearly contradicts the strict liability interpretation advanced by the Board. We conclude that (the statute) does not apply to a first time, inadvertent failure to renew a license.[23]

Thus, Nurse Sande's failure to renew her license was not a willful and repeated violation of the Nurse Practice Act and therefore reversed the decision of the Board of Nursing.

C. Substance Abuse

Impaired nurses constitute the most prevalent category of disciplinary actions. Courts are unlikely to reverse decisions to take action against a nurse's license where alcohol or drugs are involved unless there is an extreme lack of substantial evidence to support the decision. However, in the large majority of States, nurses can voluntarily enroll in rehabilitation programs without threat of formal disciplinary actions.

---

22 *Id.* at 267.

23 *Id.* at 268.

The Arkansas State Board of Nursing suspended the license of Susan Bohannon for three years for being habitually intemperate or addicted to the use of habit-forming drugs and guilty of unprofessional conduct.[24]

An investigator for the Arkansas Department of Health testified that on July 1, 1992, the Director of Pharmacy at Bates Memorial Hospital submitted seven vials of Demerol for quantitative analysis. All seven vials were obtained from the Emergency Department controlled drug supply; all were found to be adulterated. Audit procedures were implemented at the hospital. On July 7th, the pharmacy director found three vials of Demerol from a medicine cart on the Medical/Surgical Unit that appeared to have been tampered with in the same manner as those from the Emergency Department. These vials were submitted for testing, and one vial was adulterated.

Hospital records and testimony from Salena Wright, Nurse Manager of the Emergency Department, was that Nurse Bohannon worked in the Emergency Department at Bates Memorial Hospital until June 30, 1992, at which time she was transferred to the Medical/Surgical Unit. Nurse Bohannon was transferred because she was not performing well and was having problems getting along with physicians and other nurses. Hospital records indicated that Nurse Bohannon was the only employee to sign out Demerol in the Emergency Department and the Medical/Surgical Unit on the dates in question.

Nurse Wright testified that Nurse Bohannon was assigned to care for patient D.D. just before she resigned from Bates Memorial Hospital. D.D. came to the Emergency Department with acute abdominal pain and was given an injection of Demerol. D.D. was admitted to the Medical/Surgical Unit at 5:00 a.m. on July 6th, free of pain. Nurse Wright cared for D.D. and charted she was pain-free throughout the day. Nurse Bohannon took over the care of D.D. at 7:00 p.m. on July 6th. On July 7th, Nurse Bohannon charted an injection of Demerol at 7:50 p.m. on July 6th and at 5:00 a.m. on July 7th. When asked if she had received anything for pain, D.D. told Nurse Wright that she had complained of a headache and received two pills, but that was all.

After this incident, Nurse Wright did a retrospective review of other patients for whom Nurse Bohannon had cared. She found that Nurse Bohannon had cared for another patient on July 1st who had been unresponsive. Although there was no change in the patient's condition, the medication administration charts signed by Nurse Bohannon reflected that she gave Demerol at 8:10 p.m. on July 1st, and again at 2:00 a.m., 3:00 a.m., and 6:00 a.m. on July 2nd. There was no indication of irritability or restlessness of the patient to warrant pain medication. It was also noted this was the only Demerol the patient received throughout her stay at the hospital.

---

24 *Bohannon v. Arkansas State Board of Nursing*, 895 S.W.2d 923 (Ark. 1995).

Nurse Bohannon had been very candid about being a recovering substance abuser when she applied for a position at the hospital and agreed to submit to random drug tests. On July 7th, Nurse Bohannon was asked to submit to a drug test. At first, Nurse Bohannon agreed, but became increasingly agitated and irritated, and stated that she thought she was "set up." After three trips to the bathroom in a supposedly unsuccessful attempt to collect a urine specimen, Nurse Bohannon refused to take the test and stated that she was resigning from her employment.

After hearing extensive testimony, the Board concluded that Nurse Bohannon diverted controlled substances to herself and then falsified medical records to reflect the drugs had been given to patients at both Bates Memorial Hospital and Eureka Springs Memorial Hospital (she had worked there for 21 days and evidence of substance abuse was admitted). The Board suspended her license for three years and set out conditions for reinstatement.

The court first discussed the scope of its review of the decision of the Board.

If there is any substantial evidence to support the agency's decision, the reviewing court will not reverse. Substantial evidence is valid, legal, and persuasive evidence that a reasonable mind might accept to support a conclusion and force the mind to pass beyond speculation and conjecture. To prove an absence of substantial evidence, appellant (Nurse Bohannon) must show that fair-minded persons could not reach the same conclusion. The question is not whether the testimony would have supported a contrary finding, but whether it would support the finding that was made. It is the prerogative of the agency to believe or disbelieve any witness and to decide what weight to accord the evidence. (Citations omitted.)[25]

The court concluded: (1) evidence substantially support the Board's finding that Nurse Bohannon diverted drugs from her employers at Bates Memorial Hospital and at Eureka Springs Memorial Hospital and made false documentation about those drugs at both facilities; and (2) this conduct demonstrated that Nurse Bohannon acted in an unprofessional manner. The Board's suspension of Nurse Bohannon's license for three years with conditions for reinstatement was upheld.

D. Unauthorized Practice of Medicare

Linda Weyandt, CRNA, worked at the Veterans Hospital in Houston and ran an independent clinic, Associated Hypnotherapy and Pain Management Services of Texas ("Clinic").[26] Signs at the clinic and in the yellow pages advertisement identified CRNA Weyandt to clients as "Dr. Linda J. Weyandt." An undercover police

---

25 *Id.* at 926.

26 *Weyandt v. Texas*, 35 S.W.3d 144 (Tx.App. Houston [14th District] 2000).

officer visited Nurse Weyandt's clinic. Nurse Weyandt failed to clarify that she was not licensed to practice medicine, she examined the police officer's arm, passed electrical current through it, attempted to perform hypnosis and charged the officer $75 for the visit. On a subsequent search of the clinic, police officers found a cabinet full of prescriptions drugs, including Lidocaine. A jury convicted Nurse Weyandt of practicing medicine without a license. Nurse Weyandt appealed on five grounds: (1) legal insufficiency of the evidence; (2) factual insufficiency of the evidence; (3) the trial court's decision to admit evidence of extraneous crimes; (4) the unconstitutional vagueness of the Medical Practice Act's prohibition against the unauthorized practice of medicine as it applied to her; and (5) the violation of her constitutional right to remain silent when the prosecutor inadvertently used her name when he called a witness to the stand. The relevant language of the Medical Malpractice Act provided: it shall be unlawful for any individual, partnership, trust, association, or corporation by the use of any letters, word, or terms as an affix on stationary or on advertisement, or in any other manner, to indicate that the individual, trust, association, or corporation is entitled to practice medicine if the individual or entity is not licensed to do so."[27] Nurse Weyandt argued that the words "in any other manner" did not provide adequate notice of what was prohibited. To be unconstitutionally vague, a statute either must fail to provide a reasonable person sufficient information to understand exactly what conduct is prohibited or it must provide insufficient notice of the prohibited conduct to law enforcement officers. The court concluded that the statute was not unconstitutionally vague because is prohibits the use of the initials "M.D." and "doctor" in ways that might suggest that an unlicensed individual or entity is entitled to practice medicine, which is exactly what Nurse Weyandt did here.

SECTION 5-4: COURT REVIEW OF ACTIONS

The scope of review of a Board's decision by a court is extremely limited. The appropriate constitutional standard of review is restricted to considering whether the order of the Board is supported by substantial evidence justifying the order made, whether the Board acted within the scope of its statutory authority, and whether the action of the Board was arbitrary, capricious, or unreasonable.[28]

John Wilson sought review of the decision of the Mississippi State Board of Nursing to revoke his nursing license.[29] Nurse Wilson is a 42-year-old registered nurse who was employed in 1987 as a nursing supervisor in the chemical depend-

---

27 *Id.* at 155.

28 *Scott v. State ex rel. Board of Nursing of the State of Nebraska*, 244 N.W.2d 683, 689 (Neb. 1976).

29 *Mississippi State Board of Nursing v. Wilson*, 624 So.2d 485 (Miss. 1993).

ency unit at the Mississippi State Hospital. The evidence was that Nurse Wilson was addicted to or dependent upon alcohol or other habit-forming drugs, primarily cocaine, and Nurse Wilson engaged in conduct constituting a crime and likely to deceive, defraud, or harm the public.

On January 17, 1990, Nurse Wilson appeared at a disciplinary hearing before the Board based on a complaint filed on November 16, 1989. The complaint alleged: (1) Nurse Wilson was addicted to or dependent on alcohol or other habit-forming drugs; (2) Nurse Wilson engaged in conduct constituting a crime, i.e., false pretenses; and (3) Nurse Wilson engaged in conduct likely to deceive, defraud, or harm the public. The complaint resulted from an allegation that Nurse Wilson, with the intent to defraud, fraudulently received from an employee an $80 check and converted these funds to his own use.

Nurse Wilson testified he had not used drugs or alcohol in any form since 1988 and was in after care. A urine screen in July 1990 did not detect the presence of any habit-forming drugs.

An employee testified she was asked to pay for her drug screens by Nurse Wilson although evidence was there was no charge for drug screens. Nurse Wilson admitted that he endorsed the check from the employee, deposited it in his personal account, and never reimbursed the employee.

Transcripts of prior hearings conducted before the Board on December 2, 1976, January 17, 1979, March 27, 1980, and March 26, 1981 were introduced at the hearing which reflected Nurse Wilson's prior history with habit-forming drugs. Nurse Wilson previously had stipulations placed on his nursing license which was subsequently revoked in 1980 when he was found to be "habitually intemperate" with habit-forming drugs, namely Demerol and Morphine. His nursing license was reinstated in March 1981.

In examining the scope of judicial review permitted under Mississippi law, the court noted: "The only grounds for overturning administrative agency action by the appellate process is that the state agency has acted capriciously, unreasonably, arbitrarily; has abused its discretion or has violated a vested constitutional right of a party."[30] There is a rebuttable presumption in favor of the action of the Board and the burden of proof is on the nurse challenging its action.[31]

In examining whether there was substantial credible evidence of addiction or dependency, the court noted Nurse Wilson testified that he had not used drugs or alcohol in any form since 1988, and the urine screen in July 1990 was negative for habit-forming drugs. The Board based its revocation, at least in part, on Nurse Wilson's 10 year history of addiction to or dependence upon cocaine or other habit-forming drugs. Although active addiction at the time of the hearing

---

30 *Id.* at 489.

31 *Id.*

was not required for revocation, the court reasoned that some temporal proximity of active addiction to the disciplinary action was required. "The Board's stated position that it has the power to revoke a license if it finds addiction to have been active ten years in the past, even if it is in 'full remission' . . . is simply unreasonable."[32] The court concluded the Board's finding of addiction was arbitrary, meaning "it is done without adequately determining principle; not done according to reason or judgment, but depending upon the will alone—absolute in power, tyrannical, despotic, non-rational—implying either a lack of understanding or a disregard for the fundamental nature of things."[33]

The Board's finding of fraud or conduct that was deemed quasi-criminal in nature was also discussed. In reviewing the testimony of the employee and Nurse Wilson regarding paying $80 for drug screens for which there was no charge, the court concluded that Nurse Wilson intentionally lied to the employee about the cost of the drug screens to induce her to part with her money, which she did. "There is clear and convincing evidence in the record that Wilson possessed the requisite intent to defraud the employee."[34] Thus, the Board met its burden of proof with regard to Nurse Wilson's conduct constituting a crime and likely to deceive, defraud, or harm the public. Based on the court's finding, the case was remanded to the Board of Nursing for further proceedings.

In 1991, the Director of the Illinois Department of Professional Regulation ordered Marvin Ziporyn's medical license indefinitely suspended and his controlled substance license revoked.[35] This was the result of a complaint alleging that between June 9, 1984 and February 11, 1986, Ziporyn had prescribed over 1,036,500 mg of Demoral for a patient. The complaint alleged that by so treating this patient, Ziporyn failed to exercise currently accepted standards of medical care, had prescribed a habit-forming controlled substance in a way other than for therapeutic purposes and had dispensed controlled substances other than in good faith.

Ziporyn attempted to have his medical license restored in late 1991 and again in April 1996. At the hearings regarding restoration, Ziporyn testified that: he had done nothing wrong in the first place; that he did not attend follow-up courses because he was well prepared to teach the teachers; he had not sought medical treatment, psychotherapy, or counseling since the suspension; since the time that his license was suspended, he had continued to hold himself out as a physician; and he felt that the now five year suspension of his medical license was clearly out of proportion to the infractions. Upon review by the Administrative Law Judge,

---

32 *Id.* at 492.

33 *Id.*

34 *Id.* at 494.

35 *Ziporyn v. Zollar*, 724 N.E.2d 180 (Ill. App. 1999).

the conclusion was that the "mere passage of time did not justify the restoration of his medical license."[36]

Ziporyn appealed, claiming that indefinite suspension "shocks the conscious, is unfair, unwarranted, unreasonable, excessive and disproportionate to the offense" and that the "condition that he undergo a mental and physical examination was total improper and the requirement that he take a refresher course on post-traumatic stress disorder was ludicrous."[37] The court noted that its function is to ascertain whether the findings and conclusions of the regulatory agency were against the manifest weight of the evidence. The court recognized: "The State of Illinois had the legitimate interest in regulating medical professionals in order to promote and protect the public welfare. (Cite omitted) The very purpose of licensing is to ensure professional competency for the protection of the public."[38]

The responsibility of the court is to give deference to the regulatory agency's expertise and experience; it is the regulatory agency, and not the courts, that are responsible for determining sanctions for individual cases necessary to protect the public. The probationary terms imposed by the regulatory agency had not been complied with which reflects that Ziporyn has not been rehabilitated as to warrant the public's trust, and there is evidence that his practice of psychiatry imposes danger to the public. The court agreed that Ziporyn should be required to complete the SPEX exam, a 7-hour, 350 question, computer-administered exam as it was "not arbitrary, unreasonable, and unnecessarily burdensome" in light of the evidence.

REFERENCES

Beck, J. M. and Blake, M. B., *Do's and Don'ts When the State Licensing Board Comes To Call*, 34 Greater Kansas City Medical Bulletin (March 1994).

Calfee, B., et al., *Going Before The Board: How to Prepare Yourself*, 95 Nursing 56 (March 1995).

Howard, P., *The Death of Common Sense* (1995).

Mannino, K. M., *The Nursing Shortage: Contributing Factors, Risk Implications, and Legislative Efforts To Combat The Shortage*, 15 Loyola Consumer Law Review 143 (2003).

Winn, J., *Endorsement: State v. National Licensure*, 82 Federation Bulletin 9 (1995).

---

36 *Id.* at 183.

37 *Id.* at 183–184.

38 *Id.* at 187.

CHAPTER 6

Documenting and Managing Health Information

Health information has taken on a life of its own! Given the growing complexities of the health care system and the increasing legal significance of health information, the purposes and issues related to health information, have exploded. Health information is no longer a "paper medical record," but exists in written form, on microfilm, as data, or be stored electronically. It is located in numerous entities, cities, and States.

More people want access to health information for a multitude of purposes: for continuity in the care and treatment of a patient when numerous health care providers and facilities are involved; for analysis, study and evaluation of the quality of care rendered to patients; to verify that billed services were rendered and to determine whether coverage is available. Health information is critical in prosecuting and defending malpractice claims, as well as in other legal and administrative proceedings. Health information provides clinical data for use in research and education.

With the shift of health information from paper to electronic formats, the potential for patients to access, use, and disclose sensitive personal health data has increased. Congress enacted the Health Insurance Portability and Accountability Act of 1996 (HIPAA) for several reasons to ensure health insurance coverage after leaving an employer; to provide standards for facilitating health-care-related electronic transactions; and to mandate federal privacy protections for health information. The HIPAA Privacy Rule, actually a series of federal regulations, is the first ever federal privacy standard to protect health information. The intent is to establish a uniform, federal floor of privacy protections for patients across the country. The HIPAA Privacy Rule was effective April 14, 2003. Certain small health plans have an additional year to comply. There are two other HIPAA provisions yet to become effective. The Transaction and Code Set Standards became effective on October 16, 2003; however, the federal agency overseeing HIPAA, Centers for Medicare and Medicaid Services (CMS), will not begin to enforce compliance with these regulations until further notice. The Security Rule, which further defines safeguards for health information, has a compliance date of April 2005.

As late as November 2002, hearings were held throughout the country and confirmed "an extremely high level of confusion, misunderstanding, frustration, anxiety, fear, and anger as the April 14, 2003 compliance date nears."[1] Although there was wide-spread support for the goals of the HIPAA Privacy Rule, concerns were raised because of the preemption of State laws that are more stringent than HIPAA. With no national coordination of preemption issues compliance is much more difficult, costly, and complicated. Comments that were heard included: rural providers had given up on compliance; providers would drop out of participating in Federal health care programs because they cannot afford to absorb the cost of compliance and there is no way to pass along the costs; and negative health outcomes were already occurring because of providers refusing to share patient health information and reporting of essential health data had declined. *The stage is set. . . .*

SECTION 6.1: APPLICABLE LAWS

A. Federal Privacy Rule (HIPAA)

Regulations were proposed and published by the United States Department of Health and Human Services (DHHS) in December 2000. Based on information received through public comment, testimony at public hearings and meetings at the request of health care industries and stake holders, modifications to the proposed rule were proposed in August 2002 to address unintended effects on health care quality and access. However, the significant hype and commercialism in response to the December 2000 proposed regulations caused, and continues to cause, significant confusion as to the contents of the final regulations.[2]

---

1 Letter to Secretary Thompson from John R. Lumpkin, Chair, National Committee on Vital and Health Statistics, at http://ncvhs.hhs.gov/021125lt.htm.

2 Be cautious of referring to documents that only reference the HIPAA Privacy Rule as proposed in December 2000 as there were significant modifications made in the August 2002 final regulations! A good reference for these modifications is Kansas Hospital Association, HIPAA Privacy User Guide Addendum (Jan. 2003).

Overview and Key Principles

The HIPAA Privacy Rule regulates how certain entities, called covered entities, use and disclose certain individually identifiable health information, called protected health information (PHI), and establishes key rights for patients as it relates to their health information. The HIPAA Privacy Rule does the following:

1. Gives patients more control over their health information;
2. Sets boundaries on the use and disclosure of health information;
3. Establishes appropriate safeguards to protect the privacy of health information;
4. Holds violators with civil and criminal penalties for violations of privacy rights;
5. Strikes a balance when public health responsibilities support disclosure of certain health information;
6. Enables patients to make informed choices on how individual health information may be used;
7. Enables patients to find out how their health information may be used and what disclosures have been made;
8. Generally limits release of health information to the minimum reasonably needed for the purpose of the disclosure;
9. Generally gives patients the right to obtain their own health information and to request corrections; and
10. Empowers patients to control certain uses and disclosures of their health information.

HIPAA focuses on patient protections for their health information, whether communicated orally, on paper, or in computers. HIPAA provides seven key rights to patients:

1. Right to a notice of privacy practices;
2. Right to access protected health information;
3. Right to request amended protected health information;
4. Right to request alternative means of communication PHI;
5. Right to request restrictions on PHI;
6. Right to an accounting; and
7. Right to complain about privacy practices.

By this time, the expectation is that nurses have received appropriate training on the HIPAA Privacy Rule. Training is one of the requirements under HIPAA. Vital pieces of information that you should know are: (1) what HIPAA is; (2) who your privacy officer is; (3) your level of PHI access; (4) where to get a copy of your facility/organization privacy notice; (5) what to do when you see a privacy violation; and (6) that the care of the patient always comes first.

Covered Entities

The HIPAA Privacy Rules regulates covered entities. These are defined as and include health plans, health care clearing houses, and health care providers who conduct certain financial and administrative transactions (e.g., enrollment, billing, eligibility verification) electronically. Certain small health plans have an additional year to comply. Specifically excluded as covered entities are employers, life insurance companies and public agencies that delivery social security or welfare benefits. It is possible to be both a "health care provider" and a "health care plan" at the same time. To determine if you are a covered entity, Centers For Medicare and Medicaid services (CMS) has a decision tree tool at http://www.cms.gov/hipaa/hipaa2/support/tools/decisionsupport/default.asp.

While it is theoretically possible for a nurse not to trigger the HIPAA Privacy Rule (in a practice that does not engage in "covered transactions"), i.e., nothing is transmitted electronically, only cash payments are accepted by clients, and only regular mail is used), it is still recommended the nurse be HIPAA compliant as the HIPAA Privacy Rule in essence establishes minimum standards of care for the privacy and handling of patient health information. Additionally, States are likely to amend their laws to be consistent with HIPAA.

Protected Health Information (PHI)

The HIPAA Privacy Rule has several definitions of "health information." In essence, "health information" is any health information that includes 18 unique identifiers.[3] The definition of "health information" is broad; therefore, the HIPAA Privacy Rule applies to any information that relates to any care or service, past, present, or future, provided to a patient, relates to payment for the provision of health care or identifies the patient.

Psychotherapy Notes

It is noteworthy that the HIPAA Privacy Rule creates special protection for psychotherapy notes. "Psychotherapy notes" are notes recorded by a mental health care provider documenting or analyzing the contents of conversations during a counseling session *and* are maintained separately from the patient's health information.[4] The HIPAA Privacy Rule does not mandate the use of psychotherapy

---

3 45 C.F.R. § 164.514.

4 45 C.F.R. § 164.501

notes. If psychotherapy notes are maintained, don't include them in the "designated record set."

Consent/Authorization Requirements

When the HIPAA Privacy Rule was revised in August 2002, consent for use and disclosure of health information was made optional. Consent is differentiated from authorization. An authorization to use or disclose health information is only necessary in the following situations: (1) to release the health information to the patient or the patient's authorized representative; (2) to release health information to a third party who is not otherwise authorized to receive the health information; and (3) to release psychotherapy notes.[5]

Required Forms and Policies

·A key requirement under the HIPAA Privacy Rule is that covered entities must create a form called "Notice of Privacy Practices." In effect, this creates the process whereby patients are informed about how their health information is used and disclosed. The essence of the Notice of Privacy Practices is that is constitutes informed consent for patients about their health information, information which typically has not been provided to patients. The Notice of Privacy Practices is given to patients at or prior to the first contact. It must also be posted in a clear and prominent location where patients can read it.[6] The Notice of Privacy Practices may be sent via e-mail if the patient agrees to receive it in that format. It must also be posted on any websites that provide any information about the nurse, the services provided by the nurse, or the facility/organization with which the nurse is connected. Policies required under the HIPAA Privacy Rule include: accounting of disclosures; the process for handling patient complaints, what constitutes the designated record set; minimum necessary restrictions; and how to handle patient requests to amend their health information.

Investigations and Enforcement

DHHS has designated the Office for Civil Rights (OCR) to oversee and enforce the HIPAA Privacy Rule. The OCR has been extremely diligent in providing guidance and technical assistance materials on its Website.[7] The Website

---

5 The specific requirements for the authorization required by the HIPAA Privacy Rule are set forth at 45 C.F.R. § 164.508.

6 There are numerous samples of Notice of Privacy Practices. However, your Notice must be reflective of what you do and how you do it. Assistance from the Office of Civil Rights is also available at http://www.hhs.gov/ocr/hipaa/assist.html.

7 http://www.hhs.gov/ocr/hipaa/assist.html; the OCR has received reports that some consultants and education providers have claimed that their materials or systems are endorsed or

includes an extensive, searchable collection of frequently asked questions that is continually expanded and updated. It also has a toll-free information line: 866.627.7748.

Enforcement of the HIPAA Privacy Rule by the OCR will be primarily complaint driven. The HIPAA Privacy Rule provides civil and criminal penalties for covered entities that misuse health information. For civil violations, the OCR may impose monetary penalties up to $100 per violation, up to $2,500 per year, for each requirement or prohibition violated. Criminal penalties for knowingly obtaining protected health information in violation of the law can result in $50,000 and one year in prison for certain offenses; up to $100,000 and up to 5 years in prison if the offenses are committed under "false pretenses"; and up to $250,000 and 10 years in prison if the offenses are committed with the intent to sell, transfer, or use protected health information for commercial advantage, personal gain or malicious harm.

As of September 2003, the OCR has received more than 1800 complaints of potential violations of the HIPAA Privacy Rule.[8] The majority of these complaints are simple misunderstandings of how the Privacy Rule is intended to work. Nearly thirty percent of those complaints have already been closed by the OCR because the alleged incident took place prior to the effective date of the HIPAA Privacy Rule. Others have been closed because the activities prompting the complaint did not involve covered entities. Many of the complaints submitted for what was believed to be a violation of the HIPAA Privacy Rule become used in the OCR's "Frequently Asked Questions" section on its Website. To date, there have been no civil monetary penalties imposed nor have there been any onsite visits.

The OCR is committed to pursuing a voluntary compliance approach and is using its staff to provide technical assistance to help covered entities correct violations. Only when a covered entity is unwilling to cooperate or recalcitrant will the OCR impose a civil monetary penalty.

The primary problem noted by the OCR is that patients are more affected by overzealous attempts to comply with the HIPAA Privacy Rule then they are by violations of it. In one case, doctors learned after performing a heart transplant that the donated organ might have been infected. Although they requested the donor's health information, the hospital refused to release it. Thus, they were

---

required by DHHS or OCR when DHHS and OCR have not endorsed any consultants, seminars, materials, or systems and have not certified any persons or products that's "HIPAA compliant." If you believe anyone is making false or misleading representations in regard to HIPAA training and compliance, please notify the OCR at ocrcomplaint@hhs.gov.

8 Tokraski, K., *Privacy Complaints Reflect Misunderstandings of Rule*, Medscape Medical News (September 16, 2003), at http://www.medscape.com/viewarticle/461622.

forced to treat the transplant recipient without knowing the cause of the potential infection.[9]

There have been similar scenarios throughout the country. At the Greater Baltimore Medical Center, cancer patients are waiting hours for chemotherapy treatments because of missing paperwork. A patient who was diagnosed with coronary disease was sent to a physician for a stress test; however, the referring doctor's office refused to fax the patient's health information even after receiving the patient's consent (which was unnecessary) because they were unsure that the process was secure. Labs are reticent to fax health information for fear of violating HIPAA.[10]

B. Federal Transactions and Code Set Standards

The second phase of HIPAA is the Transactions and Code Set Standards (TCS Standards). The initial compliance date was October 16, 2002, which was extended for a year by President Bush. The Centers for Medicare and Medicaid Services (CMS), the enforcement agency for TCS Standards compliance, stated recently that it will not penalize noncompliance with the Standards because of the delays caused by modifying certain portions of the regulations. CMS also will take into account the numerous obstacles to implement the TCS Standards and will work with covered entities through corrective action plans rather than penalize their noncompliance.[11]

The transactions covered by the TCS Standards include:

- Professional/institutional claims;

- Health care payment and remittance advice;

- Health claims status;

- Health care eligibility benefit inquiry;

- Health plan premium payments; and

- Referral certification and authorization.

Substantial benefits to be gained in using electronic transactions are predicted to be: (1) fifty five percent reduction in claims denials arising from client-eligibility issues; (2) fifty percent drop in staff time spent in resolving claims issues with the insurer; (3) seventy five percent reduction in referral-

---

9 Wiebe, C., *Medical Privacy Protection Still Uneven*, Medscape Medical News (May 19, 2003), at http://www.medscape.com/viewarticle/455834.

10 *Id.*

11 Yennie, H., *Your Next HIPAA Deadline: Transactions and Code Set Compliance*, Behavioral Health Management 35 (May/June 2003).

processing time; and (4) more than fifty percent drop in time spent by staff in verifying eligibility.[12]

C. Security Rule

The HIPAA Security Rule requires many standards and implementation specifications regarding electronic protected health information (PHI). Its focus is on technical controls, policies, procedures, and the need for a formal risk management program. It does not specify physical security standards or implementation specifications for *non-electronic* PHI.

The final Security Rule was issued on February 13, 2003; however, covered entities have until 2005 to comply. The key security elements are:

- Technology neutrality, reasonableness and scalability;

- "Must have" standards including security leadership and risk assessment, policies, and procedures;

- Administrative, physical, and technical standards that covered entities must address and respond to appropriately;

- Security of electronic data "in motion" and "at rest;" and

- Risk assessment analyzing risks, liabilities, cost, and benefits.

D. State Laws and HIPAA Preemption

Probably the most troublesome aspect of HIPAA is the deference given to State laws to allow them to retain some control over health information. This is "preemption," which means States laws that provide less protection than HIPAA for health information must then follow the HIPAA Privacy Rule. The difficulty is that this prevents having a single and uniform standard for health information across the country, a primary purpose of HIPAA. Thus, the Federal floor for managing health information that was the intent of Congress now has holes.

Another problematic aspect of the HIPAA Privacy Rule is that it only applies to covered entities. For non-covered entities, the individual State laws will continue to apply.

Much is being written about interpreting the HIPAA Privacy Rule and how to conduct State law preemption analyses. The result is as many different interpretations as the people who write about the subject! Thus, the HIPAA Privacy Rule is truly in its infancy stage.

---

12 For a copy of the Implementation Guide and related documents, visit http://www.wpc-edi.com/hipaa/hipaacombguides.asp or http://www.wedi.org/snip/public/articles/hipaaglossary.pdf.

The HIPAA Privacy Rule identifies four instances in which State laws will prevail: (1) State law has been the subject of a determination by the Secretary of DHHS in which the State law was held *not* to be preempted; (2) the State law is *"more stringent"* than the HIPAA Privacy Rule; (3) State law provides for the *reporting* of disease, "injury, child abuse, birth, or death, or to conduct a public health surveillance, investigation, or intervention; or (4) State law governs accessibility to, or the reporting of information in the possession of *health plans*.

Any State laws that fall into one of these four exceptions is therefore "saved" from preemption. This will generally include laws in categories 1, 3 and 4. It is the second category that will be the core of contention in attempting to decide what is "more stringent" and whether the State law is "contrary to" the HIPAA Privacy Rule. Watch for further developments. . . .

SECTION 6-2: CONTENT

Your credibility is in your recorded health information as a nurse. In malpractice actions, the verdict is usually dependent upon *who* the jurors believe, which results from what evidence they view as being the most credible. Recorded health information is perceived by jurors as the most credible evidence; it can be the best defense you have. Alternatively, the lack of credible documentation will be your demise.

It goes without saying that one of the most challenging realities faced by nurses is the documentation of patient care. It is equally evident that documentation is often considered one of the least liked nursing activities. Documentation has assumed attention from a variety of people: what is the relationship between quality of health care and patient outcomes; was the hospitalization and treatment of the patient medically necessary to justify reimbursement; were Federal conditions of participation met with the content; were entries made legally and in the normal course of business to justify admission in a legal action. More often than not, nurses are competent, delivering care within the requisite standards, but are having to defend apparent incompetency because of the poor quality of the recorded health information.

One study estimates that every hour of patient care generates another thirty to sixty minutes of paperwork for nurses.[13] Frequently nurses are working overtime to complete the necessary paperwork. Another study estimates fifteen percent to twenty percent of nurses' time is spent documenting patient information and that documentation is the most common reason for overtime.[14] Documentation of nurs-

---

13 Pricewaterhouse Coopers, *Patients or Paperwork: The Regulatory Burden Facing America's Hospitals,* Commissioned by the American Hospital Association (2001).

14 Moody, L. and Snyder, P. E., *Hospital Provider Satisfaction With The New Documentation System*, 13 Nursing Economics 24 (1995).

ing care is the foremost source of reference and communication between nurses and other health care providers, and facilitates continuity of high quality care more than anything else.

A. Why Document?

The fundamental principle regarding documentation is that if an observation or action is not charted, it is as if it did not occur. While this does not prevent a nurse from testifying regarding uncharted information, it is very easy to attack a nurse's credibility that certain events or thoughts can be recalled several years after the fact. Thus, it is equally as important to document negative findings as it is the positive findings.

Documentation must also reflect exactly what is meant. The following are some examples of documentation which hopefully are *not* accurate:

> "By the time he was admitted, his rapid heart had stopped, and he was feeling better."

> "After consultation, Dr. Doe felt we should sit tight on the abdomen and I agreed."

> "The pelvic exam was done on the floor."

> "Patient has chest pain if she lies on her side for over a year."

> "On the second day, the painful knee was better, and on the third day it had completed disappeared."

A second purpose for documentation is to obtain reimbursement for the health care facility. The amount of reimbursement is directly dependent upon the documentation in the medical records. It must reflect that all medical orders were carried out adequately and correctly, and it must reflect the results of those orders. Additionally, nurses are responsible for making diagnoses of other conditions that may require a patient to remain in the facility for a longer period of time. Frequently nurses will identify complications or additional problems that adversely affect the patient's ability to get well, be adequately taught, or be ready for discharge. Denials for reimbursement commonly arise because of the lack of documentation in the medical record, not because of the lack of justification.

The third purpose for documentation is to create a legal record for the patient. The medical record consists of important information that needs to be permanently retained for the benefit of the patient as well as for the health care providers and facility. As a legal document, it may be utilized for multiple purposes, and therefore its comprehensiveness and accuracy are imperative.

Prior to undertaking care of a patient, the nurse is responsible for reviewing the medical record to obtain adequate information about the patient's status.

A nurse cannot merely rely upon a verbal report but must spend time reviewing the medical record. Accountability will be placed on the nurse for any information contained in the medical record, not only for that information which is communicated verbally. This applies in all health care settings.

Similarly, nurses are responsible for documenting information in the medical record that is important for other health care providers in their care and treatment of the patient. This does not preclude verbal communication of certain information because of its urgency. However, verbal communication does not relieve a nurse of the responsibility for documenting the information in the medical record.

B. How To Document

The four key criteria regarding documentation are the same today as they always have been:

1. Factual information;
2. Timeliness;
3. Legibility; and
4. Approved abbreviations.

Factual information means objective information; information within the personal knowledge of the nurse who documents that information. If a nurse documents what is seen, heard, or done by someone else, the source of that information must be reflected. Otherwise, the nurse documenting assumes responsibility for the events documented.

Documenting objectively is also avoiding opinions or characterizations of events, unless the bases for those subjective interpretations are included. Make certain the "opinion" doesn't become the "fact." A common example is the entry, "Patient fell out of bed." It is extremely rare for a patient to be directly observed falling out of bed; rather, a nurse hears a loud noise from the patient's room, upon entering the room finds the patient on the floor at the side of the bed, and the patient tells the nurse: "I needed to go to the bathroom. I thought I could do it without any assistance so I tried to crawl over the end of the bed. My leg got caught and I fell." The factual and objective documentation is: "A loud noise was heard from the patient's room. Patient found on floor at the side of the bed. Patient stated: 'I needed to go to the bathroom. I thought I could do it without any assistance so I tried to crawl over the end of the bed. My leg got caught and I fell.'" Documenting that the patient fell out of bed is the nurse's *opinion* as to the events and, therefore, constitutes subjective charting.

Documentation must be timely; activities should be as time specific as possible and applicable; and information is entered into the permanent system/record as soon as practicable. Time-specific charting requires relating each patient activity to the time period when it occurred. Whether that time period is a minute, an hour, or a day will depend on the health care setting and the importance of the activity. Sometimes it is important to document specific times that events occurred, such as telephone calls to physicians, a patient's sudden change in vital signs or condition, or patient activities. The more specific the time frame in which activities can be identified, the more accurate the record. Specific timing of events can also be a critical factor in the course of litigation.

Promptly record events in the permanent source for the health information so other health care providers who have responsibility for that patient's care are knowledgeable. Because it is not always known when another health care provider may be involved with that patient, make special efforts to timely document that information which would be of extreme significance for other health care providers.

Legibility is less of a concern today with the increased use of forms and electronic communications. But illegible paper entries create negative impressions of the author, and can frustrate jurors who are trying to read it.

Abbreviations used must be approved by the health care facility. This is a requirement of the Joint Commission on Accreditation of Healthcare Organizations and many State laws. If an abbreviation cannot be interpreted by a subsequent health care provider, then harm may occur to a patient as a result.

While countersigning an entry doesn't imply that you performed the procedure, it does represent that you reviewed the entry, believe it's accurate, agree with it, and approved the care planned or given. Don't countersign unless legally required to, such as for purposes of reimbursement. If countersigning is to reflect that care is being supervised, make a separate entry of a personal assessment of or other interactions with the patient.

When required to countersign an entry, make certain that the entry is accurate, that it clearly identifies who performed any assessments and procedures, and that all pertinent information is contained in the entry. If the entry suggests that there are any problems or concerns that need to be followed up, make certain that the appropriate actions are initiated.

When and how corrections and additions can be made to health information is typically defined by policy, and perhaps State law. They must be made as required to protect the integrity of the health information.

The general recommendation to delete an entry is to draw a single line through the entry without obliterating what is written. There is no purpose for obliteration and it only raises an inference that something was written that was not intended to be read by a judge or a jury. The initials of the person making the correction, the date, and the time of the correction need to be documented by the correction to avoid *any* question about a correction being made subsequent to a potential claim or lawsuit.

The correct information is then recorded. If the correction or addition of new information occurs subsequent to the initial entry, the date and time of the new entry is indicated. Within the context of the entry, reference is made to the date and time to which the information refers. If it is appropriate, document a brief explanation of why the correction is being made.

C. Incident Reports

Incident reports record the occurrence of or potential for unusual or adverse events involving patients. They communicate the risk for a claim to risk management personnel, health care administrators, insurance carriers, and attorneys. At times they identify problems or risks to patients, a need to revise policies, or assess performance of individual health care providers.

The confidentiality and discoverability of incident reports is determined by State law, which is quite varied. To prevent an incident report from being disclosed if State law protects it as a privileged document, it must be created in a specific manner and its confidentiality maintained. Know how to complete and use incident reports.

The fact that an incident report has been completed should not be recorded with the patient's health information. However, document the events of the incident if they are important to patient care and treatment. Caution: make certain that any information documented is objective, not opinions or characterization of events.

D. Types of Documentation Systems

The impossible has been attempted: develop the "perfect nursing documentation system." To date, that has not happened—or at least I don't know about it! ("Failure is not an option!"—NASA) Current documentation systems are certainly an improvement on how nurses have traditionally documented. The primary goals are a balance act: having the most comprehensive and effective documentation system to benefit patient care; having a system that is time efficient; and having a system that is defensible in a legal action.

When implementing a new documentation system, ensure that *all* nursing personnel are adequately oriented and provided ongoing support. Many problems arise because of the complexity of the documentation system and nurses not being adequately trained. These complex systems are also especially problematic for float or agency nurses who are unfamiliar with them and don't have the time to learn how to correctly use them.

Another issue with the new documentation systems is reimbursement. Some do not incorporate care plans or protocols in the permanent medical record. Many third party payors, including Medicare and Medicaid, have expressed concerns about this. In a communication received from Medicare, the following was expressed:

> As stated in HIM 15-1, Section 2304, sufficient detail for the services furnished to patients must be available for the determination of proper payment to the provider. Determination of proper payment includes claims audits as needed. Without access to . . . protocols, it is not possible to trace charges and perform a claims audit. Furthermore, a system that requires an enormous amount of checking back and forth between various records and protocols in order to conduct an audit is not reasonable. The provider is required to maintain audible records and the medical record should be complete and able to stand alone without reference to other documents. Unauditable records will be denied.[15]

Flowsheets are now common in lieu of narrative notes. These arguably provide a better mechanism for comprehensive assessment of patients, while requiring less time to document. However, flowsheets do not eliminate the need for some narrative charting. Learn how these two documentation tools can compliment each other without duplicating information charted.

In using flowsheets, the key criteria to make them accurate and legally defensible are:

1. Fill in all blanks or write "N/A;"
2. Note the specific time or a limited time frame for the assessment or activity;
3. Make certain it is clear who performed the assessment or activity;
4. The patient's name and date must be on each flowsheet or page of a multi-page document; and
5. If initials are used, the provider's full name and credentials must be written on the page.

Charting-by-exception is another form of documenting. There are many variations of this system, and frequently documentation as required by this system is inconsistent at facilities. It also challenges the legal maxim: "If it was not charted, then it was not done."

---

15 *Personal Communication* (August 1991).

In *Lama v. Borras*,[16] the Appellate Court upheld the jury's conclusion that the Hospital was negligent in using the "charting-by-exception" method of recording notes in the patient's medical record.

Romero Lama was suffering from back pain, and was referred to Dr. Borras, a neurosurgeon. Mr. Lama had surgery on April 9, at which time Dr. Borras discovered an extruded disc and attempted to remove the extruded material. Either because Dr. Borras failed to remove the material or operated at the wrong level, Mr. Lama's symptoms returned several days after the operation. A second operation was performed on May 15th. Dr. Borras did not order antibiotics pre-operative or post-operative.

On May 17th, a nurse's note indicates that the bandage covering Mr. Lama's surgical wound was "very bloody," a symptom indicating infection. On May 18th, Mr. Lama experienced pain at the site of the incision, another symptom consistent with an infection. On May 19th, the bandage was "soiled again." According to the court, "a more complete account of Mr. Lama's evolving condition is not available because the Hospital instructed nurses to engage in 'charting by exception,' a system whereby nurses did not record qualitative observations for each of the day's three shifts, but instead made such notes only when necessary to chronicle important changes in a patient's condition."[17]

On the night of May 20th, Mr. Lama experienced severe discomfort in his back. On May 21st, Dr. Piazza diagnosed the problem as discitis and initiated antibiotics. Discitis is extremely painful and very slow to cure; Mr. Lama was hospitalized for several additional months while undergoing treatment for the infection.

Mr. Lama filed a lawsuit against Dr. Borras and the Hospital, alleging the Hospital: (1) failed to prepare, use, and monitor proper medical records; and (2) failed to provide proper hygiene at the hospital premises.

At trial, testimony was given that a regulation of the Puerto Rico Department of Health, required qualitative nurses' notes for each nursing shift. There was no dispute that during Mr. Lama's hospitalization, the nurses did not prepare the required notes for every shift, but instead followed the Hospital's Policy, "Charting-By-Exception." The Hospital argued that it didn't know whether the nurses observed, but failed to record, any material symptoms that would have led the physician to investigate the infection at an earlier stage. The Hospital's position was that even under the "Charting By Exception" Policy, nurses regularly recorded such information as the patient's temperature, vital signs, and medications.

---

16   16 F.3d 473 (1st Cir. 1994).

17   *Id.* at 475–476.

Yet, additional trial evidence reflected that as part of the practice of charting-by-exception, nurses did not regularly record certain information important to the diagnosis of an infection, such as the changing characteristics of the surgical wound and the patient's complaints of post-operative pain. One former nurse at the Hospital who took care of Mr. Lama testified that, under the "Charting-By-Exception" Policy, she would not report a patient's pain if she either did not administer any medicine or simply gave the patient an aspirin-type medication as opposed to a narcotic.

Additional evidence by the plaintiff's expert witness was that Mr. Lama's records contained scattered signs of infection that deserved further investigation, such as an excessively bloody bandage and local pain at the site of the wound. The conclusion was that Mr. Lama acquired a wound infection as early as May 17th when the nurse noted the very bloody bandage, or possibly May 19th, when Mr. Lama complained of pain at the site of the wound. The wound infection then developed into discitis on or about May 20th when Mr. Lama began experiencing excruciating back pain. Although the initial infection may not have been preventable, the key question is whether early detection and treatment of the infection would have prevented the infection from reaching the disc innerspace in the critical period prior to May 20th. Plaintiff's expert witness testified that "time is an extremely important factor" in handling an infection; a twenty-four hour delay in treatment can make a difference; and a delay of several days carries a high risk that the infection will not be properly controlled."[18]

As the court concluded:

> As to Hospital del Maestro, it was entirely possible for the jury to conclude that the particular way in which the medical and nursing records were kept constituted evidence of carelessness in monitoring the patient after the second operation. Perhaps the infection would have been reported and documented earlier. Perhaps the hospital was negligent in not dealing appropriately with wound inspection and cleaning, (and) bandage changing . . ."[19]

It was the Hospital's "substandard record-keeping procedures (that) delayed the diagnosis and treatment of Romero's wound infection at a time when controlling the wound infection was likely to prevent the development of the more serious discitis."[20] The court, therefore, upheld the jury verdict awarding the plaintiff $600,000 in compensatory damages.

---

18 *Id.* at 481.

19 *Id.* at 477.

20 *Id.* at 481.

In this case, conditions that deviated from the norm for Mr. Lama were not documented, which is required even under the charting-by-exception system. But it is also evident that the system makes it difficult to prove the attentiveness of the nursing staff and creates an adverse inference for the jury. As health care standards and documentation systems evolve and change, they will have to be clearly explained to the jury to demonstrate that the standards of care have been met.

A survey conducted in a 1,000 bed long-term care institution, which encompasses three previously autonomous facilities, evaluated different types of documentation systems. The records were reviewed with the main objective of assessing the quality of the information nurses documented about the care they provided. The documentation systems used were narrative, charting by exception, "fill in the blanks," and check lists. The data reflected that nursing assessments were performed in 94% of the records; however, there were differences with respect to the time these assessments were completed. The audit reflected that nurses placed more emphasis on making patient assessments and arriving at nursing diagnoses than evaluating their interventions and patient outcomes. It was noted that one explanation for the just over 50% of records reflecting patient status on a continuous basis was that the documentation system in that facility, was charting-by-exception. It was further noted that the level of progress in resolving patient's medical problems was not readily identifiable, nor was their current health status. There was also duplicating and time consuming aspects of the documentation systems.[21]

SECTION 6-3: ELECTRONIC COMMUNICATIONS

Technology has evolved such that health information is recorded and transmitted in many different forms: paper; Internet; electronic data; e-mails; and cellular telephones. The Electronic Communications Privacy Act (ECPA) was amended in 1986 in response to the need to protect these new forms of electronic communications.[22] The ECPA defines "electronic communication" as "any transfer of signs, signals, writing, images, sounds, data, or intelligence of any nature transmitted in whole or in part by a wire, radio, electromagnetic, photoelectronic, or photooptical system that affects interstate or foreign commerce . . ."[23] It also provides that no otherwise privileged wire, oral, or electronic communication intercepted either

---

21 Martin, A., et al., *Documentation Practices of Nurses in Long-Term Care*, 8 J. Clinical Nursing 345 (1991).

22 18 U.S.C. §§ 2510–2521, 2701–2711.

23 18 U.S.C. § 2510(12).

illegally or in accordance with one of the statutorily recognized exceptions shall lose its privileged character.[24]

Because of the increased flow of health information through electronic means, the liability potentials have increased. Employees, Medical Staff members, volunteers, and students may inappropriately use e-mails or have access to protected e-mail. The Internet is used as a medical library, offering advice and even consultation. In 1999, 83.3 million Americans accessed the Internet.[25]

What is now being referred to as "E-Health" is quickly having a tremendous impact on health care. "E-Health is defined as the emerging field in the intersection of medical informatics, public health, and business that refers to health services and information delivered or enhanced through the Internet and related technologies."[26] What this reflects is a change in how we think about health care and look to improve it—by using information and communication technology. Many health care facilities now have electronic medical records (EMR), sometimes also referred to as computer-based patient records (CPR). These electronic systems encourage a complete integration of all health information related to a patient with easier access to health care providers.

The American Medical Association developed Guidelines for physician-patient electronic communications.[27] These Guidelines emphasize that these new electronic communications should not replace but enhance interpersonal contacts with patients. We are just beginning to see the legal effects of electronic communications, including whether and how they will be admissible in legal actions.

In *Linnen v. A.H. Robins Company, Inc.*[28], plaintiffs filed a wrongful death action and requested the production of any e-mail messages retained by Wyeth-Ayerst Laboratories, one of the defendants. Wyeth objected to this discovery request as it would require them to restore backup tapes containing the e-mail messages which would be unduly burdensome and costly. In fact, the motion was characterized as a "multi-million dollar fishing expedition," and Wyeth argued that other documents responsive to the request had already been produced. The court noted that these tapes had the potential to contain relevant material that the plaintiff should have the opportunity to examine. A discovery request aimed at the production of records retained in an electronic form is no

---

24 18 U.S.C. § 2510(4).

25 Dobbins, P., *Provision of Legal and Medical Services on the Internet: Licensure and Ethical Considerations*, 3 North Carolina J. of Law and Tech. 353 (Spring 2002).

26 Guilick, P.G., *E-Health and Future of Medicine: The Economic, Legal, Regulatory, Cultural, and Organizational Obstacles*, 12 Albany L. J. of Science and Tech. 351 (2002).

27 http://www.ama-asn.org/ama/pub/printcat/2386.html.

28 *Linnen v. A.H. Robins Company, Inc.*, 1999 WL 462015 (Mass. Sup. 1999).

different from a request for documents contained in an office file cabinet. Although it may require more sophisticated equipment to restore them, they certainly are discoverable. As the court noted: "This is one of the risks taken on by companies which have made the decision to avail themselves of the computer technology now available to the business world."[29]

Plaintiffs also argued that Wyeth intentionally destroyed backup tapes of e-mails that were responsive to plaintiff's request for production of documents and had been the subject of an ex parte order requiring defendant to preserve these documents. The Court agreed that it was undisputed that Wyeth had failed to preserve electronic mail backup tapes as required by the court, and agreed that this was inexcusable conduct on the part of Wyeth. The Court agreed that at the time of trial, the jury would be instructed that an adverse inference may be drawn from the fact that documents were destroyed by Wyeth, a concept known as the "spoliation inference." This permits the jury to infer that the party who destroyed potentially relevant evidence did so out of a realization that the evidence was infavorable. The Court further ordered Wyeth to pay the costs and fees associated with the plaintiff's efforts to pursue this discovery including several depositions and that Wyeth reimburse the plaintiffs for the fees and costs incurred by their attorneys as a result of this issue.

Law has also been established that data in computerized form is discoverable even if paper hard copies of the information have been produced and that the producing party can be required to design a computer program to extract the data from its computerized records.[30]

The issue of the admissibility of computer printouts of system data addressed by the Maine Supreme Court in *United Airlines, Inc. v. Hewins Travel Consultants, Inc.*[31] Hewins argued that the computer records were inadmissible summaries. The Court noted that the computer records in question are originals of the usage data stored on the computer tape and are admissible pursuant to the pertinent rule of evidence: "If data are stored in a computer or similar device, any printout or other output readable by sight, shown to reflect the data accurately, is an original."[32] Hewins then attempted to argue that the records were not admissible because they were made years after the data was entered and in preparation for litigation, and therefore not as part of regularly conducted business. The Court held that Hewins was improperly focusing on the time of printing the computer records rather than the entry of the raw data

---

29 *Id.* at 6.

30 *Anti-Monopoly, Inc. v. Hasbro, Inc.*, 958 F.Supp. 895 (S.D.N.Y. 1997), *affirmed*, 130 F.3d 1101 (2nd Cir. N.Y. 1997), *cert. denied*, 525 U.S. 813 (U.S. 1998).

31 *United Airlines, Inc. v. Hewins Travel Consultants, Inc.*, 622 A.2d 1163 (Me. 1993).

32 Fed.R. Evid. 1001(3).

which was entered at or near the time of the event recorded and in the normal course of business. As recognized by the Nebraska Supreme Court, a printout made in preparation for trial "exalts the form over the substance. The retrieval from the taped record . . . was made for the purpose of the trial, but the taped record and the information and calculations thereon were made in the usual course of business and for the purpose of the business alone."[33]

An issue with the admissibility of electronic communications is the extent of the foundation required to make it admissible as a legal document. In *United States v. Koontz*[34], the defendant argued that a computer-generated booking report from an Iowa jail showing what time an individual was released from jail was inappropriately admitted. The Eighth Circuit disagreed, stating "We see no reason to reject the booking report simply because it was computer-generated."[35]

The general rule for computer business records to be admissible requires: (1) they are kept pursuant to a routine procedure designed to ensure their accuracy; (2) they are created for motives that intend to assure accuracy; and (3) that they are not themselves merely accumulations of hearsay.[36] Some courts have held that it is not necessary to present testimony regarding the mechanical accuracy of the computer which generated the record, nor is it necessary that the individual who programmed the computer testify to authenticate the computer-generated records.[37]

Electronic health information expands the potential for how patient privacy can be breached or how the integrity of patient information can be lost. The goals are too narrow and limit the threats to the security and integrity of this information. Key elements include a privacy and security policy, management controls to implement and enforce the policy, appropriate technical safeguards, proper system maintenance and support, and disaster recovery capabilities. Health care providers should also have effective mechanisms to protect electronic health information from:

1. Unauthorized disclosure to personnel;
2. Unauthorized disclosure to outsiders;
3. Accidental errors;
4. Malicious errors;

---

33 *Transport Indemnity v. Seib*, 132 N.W.2d 871, 875 (Neb. 1965).

34 *United States v. Koontz* ,143 F.3d 408 (8th Cir. 1998).

35 *Id.* at 412. (Defendant's argument was not persuasive because there was no case law cited in support of his contention.)

36 *Trans-Rim Enterprises Ltd. v. Adolph Corps.* Company, 52 F.3d 338 (10th Cir. 1995).

37 *United States v. Salgado*, 250 F.3d 438 (6th Cir. 2001), *cert. denied*, 122 S. Ct. 306 (2001).

5. Temporary loss of health information; and

6. Destruction of health information.

Risks must be identified, planned for, and appropriately managed. The parameters to focus on include:

1. Identifying what can go wrong with the system or how it may malfunction;

2. Minimizing the malfunction;

3. Identifying the consequences of system failure; and

4. Mitigating those consequences.

The failures of an electronic health information system may be obvious or non-obvious. An obvious failure occurs where the system does not operate at all. A non-obvious failure includes incomplete or incorrect output which may be due to human operator failure, incorrect processing of the data, or intentional alteration of the data. Another non-obvious failure is the unauthorized access to or use of the data.

Multiple liabilities arise with the use of an electronic health information system. If the system is non-functioning, there may be a breach of the warranty whereby the liability is attributed to the vendor or manufacturer of the system. However, if the health care facility fails to use the system properly or to appropriately maintain the system, it will incur liability. The liability may also be defined by contract.

If the failure arises from human operator error, the operator, facility, and the person who trained the operator will be subjected to liability. Any *deliberate* and *willful* alteration of the data is an intentional tort. Allegations would include: lack of proper training; lack of quality control; or negligence on the part of the operator. If a nurse relies upon erroneous data in rendering care to a patient, and the nurse is sued for negligence arising from the erroneous data, the nurse could sue the facility and operator.

Unauthorized access to or use of health information violates the patient's right of privacy, which occurs if health information is at a terminal and accessed by unauthorized persons. Breaches of security may cause a court to determine that electronic health information lacks the reliability required to be admissible as evidence. Without admissibility of the health information, legal actions cannot be pursued or defended.

Security mechanisms must balance health information privacy and integrity against the need for quick and easy access to health information by those who need it, and with the design and operation required for health information to be admissible as evidence in court. The *reasonableness of* security depends upon:

1. The state of commercially available electronic technology;
2. The affordability of security technology, procedures, and techniques;
3. The likelihood that security will fail and the risk that such a failure could be intentional;
4. The magnitude of harm that could result if security fails, is inadequate, or is breached;
5. Known and reasonably anticipated threats to security;
6. Standards promulgated by nationally recognized standard-setting organizations and professional associations in the fields of health information, health care informatics, and computer security; and
7. Legal requirements concerning accessibility of patient health information.

Severe sanctions must be imposed upon employees and medical staff who access or use data for which they are not authorized, or for disclosure of access codes to non-appropriate personnel. Sanctions should likely be immediate termination or loss of medical staff privileges. Sanctions should be set forth in facility policies, bylaws, or employee personnel manuals or handbooks. Liabilities for unauthorized access to or use of data include defamation, invasion of privacy, and breach of contract.

SECTION 6-4: USE AND DISCLOSURE

A. Privacy and Confidentiality

"Privacy" and "confidentiality" are separate and distinct concepts that apply to health information. The right of privacy emanates from the Constitution as set forth by the United States Supreme Court in *Roe v. Wade*.[38] This Constitutional right is based upon the Fourteenth Amendment, which affords the rights of personal liberty and protection from intrusion into private matters.

Confidentiality is a statutory creation giving legal status to relationships with certain individuals. It was established to promote trust in professional relationships, to acknowledge respect for sensitive information, and to facilitate truthful and complete disclosure of information.

Examples of statutorily-created privileges include physician-patient, nurse-patient, psychologist-patient, clergy-patient, and attorney-client. In many states, the physician-patient privilege extends to protect health information created by a health care facility. Confidentiality is controlled by the person for or to whom

---

38 410 U.S. 113 (1973).

an individual's privacy is relinquished, i.e., the professional. This differs from privacy, which is controlled by the individual.

B. Disclosure Procedures

Health information in its original form is the property of the health care provider or facility creating it. *Copies* of health information are provided to patients and others authorized to access the health information. The health care provider/facility has the right to control how health information is released. Providers should take *reasonable* precautions to verify the authority of the person seeking access to health information as required by the HIPAA Privacy Rule.[39] *Unreasonable* restriction of access to health information can be tantamount to a refusal to release information, and result in a lawsuit for interfering with that patient right.[40] The failure to release appropriately requested health information may also result in punitive damages.[41]

Charges to make copies of health information must be reasonable and related to the actual expenses. Some States have laws limiting the amount that may be charged for copying health information. Under HIPAA, the fee must be: "reasonable, cost-based and only include costs for: (1) copying, including costs of supplies and labor for copying; (2) postage (if mailed); and (3) preparing a summary if so requested.[42]

The HIPAA Privacy Rule establishes the right of health care providers to use or to disclose health information to a patient under the following circumstances: (1) the access requested is reasonably likely to endanger the life or physical safety of the patient or another person; (2) the protected health information makes reference to another person; (3) the access requested is reasonably likely to cause substantial harm to such other persons; or (4) the request for access is made by the patient's personal representative and providing the information to such personal representative is reasonably likely to cause substantial harm to the person.[43]

The health care provider/facility may require a written authorization to release health information.[44]

---

39 45 CFR § 164.514(h).

40 *Thurman v. Crawford*, 652 S.W.2d 240 (Mo. App. 1983).

41 *Wear v. Walker*, 800 S.W.2d 99 (Mo. App. 1990); *Franklin Square Hospital v. Laubach*, 569 A.2d 693 (Md.App. 1990).

42 45 CFR § 164.524(c)(4).

43 45 CFR § 164.524(a)(3).

44 45 CFR § 164.524(b)(1). Since "consent" to use and disclose health information is deemed to be implied under the HIPAA Privacy Rule for many situations, I recommend requiring an Authorization only for : uses and disclosures specifically *requested* by a patient; uses and

The request must be acted upon no later than thirty days after it is received. The use or disclosure of the requested health information must occur within the thirty days, unless it is not maintained or accessible on site, in which case an additional thirty days are provided.[45] The access to the health information requested must be in the form or format requested by the patient, if it is readily producible, or, if not, in a readable hardcopy form; or in such other form or format as agreed to by the patient.[46]

If the patient is a minor, State laws will define certain medical care and treatment or special situations in which minors are authorized to consent, which also authorizes the minor to use and disclose personal health information related to that treatment. Otherwise, the minor's parent or legal guardian is authorized to use or disclose the minor's health information. If the minor's parents are divorced, some States prohibit the noncustodial parent from accessing or controlling the minor's health information. Verify that the person requesting the health information is the parent or the appropriate legal representative for the minor.

Under both Federal and State laws, certain health information is *required* to be or *may* be disclosed. While such disclosures vary among States, generally required is reporting of communicable diseases, seizure activity, child and elder neglect and abuse, gunshot wounds, wounds sustained during a crime or an attempted crime, and cancer. Reporting made in good faith and pursuant to the appropriate law will generally give the reporting person immunity. Failure to report if required will subject the nurse to both civil and criminal liability.

There also may be common law duty to disclose health information to prevent injury or harm to an innocent third party, referred to as a duty to warn.

C. Legal Proceedings

Disclosure of health information may be compelled by a court order or a subpoena duces tecum. The designated person must appear and testify, and bring the health information described in the order or subpoena. Subpoenas may be issued by clerks of courts and various governmental boards and commissions.

The manner of serving subpoenas duces tecum is established by State and Federal law. It may be permissible to serve them by mail, or it may be required to serve them in person. Most States require service within a specified number of days prior to the date of the required appearance. Failure to comply with a subpoena duces tecum or court order without reasonable justification is punish-

---

disclosures of *psychotherapy notes*; uses and disclosures <u>not</u> permitted by the HIPAA Privacy Rule or applicable State law.

45   45 CFR § 164.524(b)(2).

46   45 CFR § 164.524(c)(2).

able as contempt of court. If there is a reason for noncompliance, a motion to quash may be filed by an attorney on behalf of the party served.

Upon receiving a court order or subpoena duces tecum to appear and produce health information, contact the attorney or judge to determine the exact time the appearance is needed. Also, if there is a conflict with the requested date and time, frequently this can be worked out with the attorney or judge.

The HIPAA Privacy Rule establishes standards for disclosing or using health information in judicial and administrative proceedings. *Please* note that these are "permissive" disclosures, not mandatory.[47] In response to an *order* of a court or administrative agency, requested health information *may* be disclosed without the patient authorizing the disclosure. However, in response to a *subpoena, discovery requests, or other lawful process,* the requested health information can only be *disclosed after the patient has been notified* of the request and provided an opportunity to file the necessary motions to prevent its release.[48] The preferred method of disclosing health information in response to a subpoena or other lawful process is to obtain evidence of the patient's authorization to do so. In and of itself, a subpoena *does not waive* the privacy or confidentiality afforded to health information.[49]

The HIPAA Privacy Rule also provides for permissive disclosures to law enforcement officers. Permissible disclosures include: information identifying or locating a suspect, fugitive, material witness, or missing person; information about an individual who is or is suspected to be a victim of a crime; information regarding a patient's death if it is suspected to have occurred from criminal conduct; health information that constitutes evidence of criminal conduct that occurred on the premises of the covered entity; and the fact that emergency health care is being provided to a patient if it may be related to a crime.[50]

Health information is subject to search warrants. Upon receipt of a search warrant: (1) contact the appropriate person, i.e. risk manager; administrator, or criminal attorney; (2) be cordial but firm with the governmental or law official; and (3) do nothing until you are so advised by the "appropriate person." To be valid, a search warrant must:

1. Be in writing;
2. Be issued in the name of the State or applicable Federal District;
3. Be directed to a governmental or law official;

---

47 45 CFR § 164.512(e)(1).

48 45 CFR § 164.512(e)(1)(ii).

49 *Fierstein v. DePaul Health Center*, 949 S.W.2d 90 (Mo.App. E.D. 1997), *affirmed.* 24 S.W.3d 220 (Mo. App. E.D. 2000) (Hospital breached fiduciary duty of confidentiality by releasing medical records in response to a subpoena).

50 45 CFR § 164.512(f).

4. Include the time and date issued;

5. Identify the property, article, material, substance, or person in sufficient detail and particularly which is to be searched for and seized;

6. Command that the described person, place, or thing be searched;

7. Command that any of the described property, articles, materials, substance, or person found be seized, photographed, or copied; and

8. Be signed by a judge or magistrate.

The person tendering the search warrant must provide photo identification. Copy the search warrant and keep an itemized receipt obtained for all property taken. Before releasing original health information, closely scrutinize the warrant as to whether it authorizes the seizure of the original health information as opposed to photocopies. Even if original health information is described, request that copies be made instead. At a minimum, copy the original health information before relinquishing it.

Refusing to permit a valid search warrant to be executed or otherwise obstructing officials during a search can result in criminal contempt proceedings and charges.

SECTION 6.5: RETENTION

Federal or State laws establish the retention times and procedures for health information. For example, health information for Medicare/Medicaid patients must be kept the longer of five years after the filing of the cost report, or the period in which lawsuits may be filed requiring production of the information. When establishing policies regarding retention of health information, consider:

1. Federal and State laws;

2. Appropriate statutes of limitation for lawsuits where the health information would be required as evidence;

3. Medical research conducted by the health care provider;

4. Storage capabilities; and

5. Recommendations of health care and health information associations.

Health information of patients involved with medical research should be retained for an extensive period of time as lawsuits may be brought years after the research is conducted. In *Mink v. University of Chicago*, the plaintiffs brought an action in 1976 based upon experiments which occurred from 1950 through 1952.[51] The recommendation is to retain health information of patients involved in research for their anticipated life span.

---

51 460 F.Supp. 713 (N.D. Ill. 1978).

In the absence of specific State requirements for retention of health information, the recommendation is to retain health information at least one year beyond the State's statute of limitations for malpractice actions and wrongful death. In many States, because the statute of limitations is extended for minors, a longer retention period will be required. Certain accrediting bodies also have retention standards to be considered. The American Health Information Management Association (AHIMA) has recommended retention standards, a summary of Federal record retention requirements, and an analysis of State laws pertaining to retention, which are excellent resources.[52]

When health care facilities merge or close, considerations must be given to how and where health information will be retained. While some States have specific statutes or regulations governing health information when a health care facility merges or closes, even in the absence of a specific law, health care providers and facilities have a fiduciary and ethical duty to maintain health information for the appropriate time periods. Patients expect health information to be available for continuity of their care as well as for legal purposes. It is generally recommended that before health records are transferred, patients be notified and given an opportunity to obtain copies of their health information. Publishing notices in the local newspaper will accomplish this.

A. Facsimiles

With facsimile machines, critical health information is immediately available to any health care provider. Yet, they increase opportunities for breaching patient privacy. Establish procedures to adequately protect patients from unauthorized or inappropriate use or disclosure of their health information. Health information may be misdirected or intercepted by individuals to whom access is not intended or authorized. There have been newspaper headlines describing events wherein health information was inadvertently faxed to a newspaper office rather than the intended recipient.

The HIPAA Privacy Rule permits transmitting health information by fax provided that health care providers have reasonable and appropriate administrative, technical, and physical safeguards to protect the privacy of health information. For example, the sender should confirm the fax number to be used, and place the fax machine in a secure location to prevent unauthorized access to the information.[53] Verify if there are any State laws applicable to the use of facsim-

---

52 AHIMA, *Practice Brief: Retention of Health Information* (2002); The Federal and State laws regarding retention are included with this document, at http://library.ahima.org/xpedio/groups/public/documents/ahima/pub_bok1_012545.html.

53 45 CFR § 164.530(c).

ile equipment or for specific types of diseases, such as sexually transmitted diseases or mental health problems.

Users of fax machines must be properly instructed on how to handle health information. Require them to double check the recipient's fax number before pressing the send key. Some fax machines have broadcast capabilities that allow one to inadvertently broadcast numerous copies of health information to widely dispersed facsimile receiving machines.

The following is suggested language for the cover page:

> This facsimile contains health information that is confidential and privileged. It is intended only for the use of the individual or entity named above. If the reader of a facsimile is not the intended recipient or the employee or agent responsible for delivering it to the intended recipient, you are hereby on notice that you are in possession of confidential and privileged information. Any dissemination, distribution, or copying of this facsimile is strictly prohibited. If you have received this facsimile in error, please immediately notify the send by telephone and return the original facsimile to the sender at the above address via the U.S. Postal Service.

Maintain faxed documents as part of the patient's health information.

SECTION 6-6: SPECIAL TYPES OF HEALTH INFORMATION

Certain types of health information typically are afforded special protections under State or Federal laws. For such information, general medical authorizations to disclose "any and all information" are not sufficient to disclose this information; rather, the authorization must explicitly delineate the information to be disclosed.

A. Alcohol and Drug Abuse

Federal statutes and regulations afford special protections to confidentiality of alcohol and drug abuse health information.[54] The patient's identity, diagnosis, prognosis, and treatment is confidential if it occurred in any Federally-assisted program that holds itself out as providing alcohol or drug abuse diagnosis, treatment, or referral for treatment. This includes any general medical care facility that has an identified unit for alcohol or drug abuse diagnosis, treatment, or referral for treatment or that has staff whose primary function is alcohol or drug abuse diagnosis, treatment, or referral for treatment. The laws prohibit the disclosure and use of health information without specific patient consent or only under certain defined circumstances. The penalty for violating any of these laws

---

54 42 U.S.C. § 290dd-3 and § 290ee-3 and 42 C.F.R. § 2.1 et seq.

is a maximum of $500 for the first offense, and a maximum of $5,000 for each subsequent offense.

The restrictions on use and disclosure are quite broad and include any health information, whether verbal, written, or electronic, that relates to a patient who has been evaluated for or been given diagnosis or treatment for alcohol or drug abuse. Information that identified a patient as an alcohol or drug abuser, or that is obtained for the purpose of treating alcohol or drug abuse, making a diagnosis for that treatment, or making a referral for that treatment is confidential. Even the fact that a patient is present in a facility may be acknowledged only with the patient's written consent or with an authorizing court order. The only exception to the prohibition on use and disclosure is for reports made pursuant to suspected child abuse or neglect.

Any requests for health information must be responded to in a way that doesn't affirmatively reveal that the patient has been or is being diagnosed or treated for alcohol or drug abuse. Provide the requestor with the Federal regulations that restrict the disclosure of alcohol or drug abuse health information.

Disclosures or uses have to be made pursuant to a consent form that includes the following elements:

1. The specific name or general designation of the program or person permitted to make the disclosure;
2. The name or title of the individual or the name of the organization to which disclosure is to be made;
3. The name of the patient;
4. The purpose of the disclosure;
5. How much and what kind of information is to be disclosed;
6. The signature of the patient, or the signature of a person authorized to give consent;
7. The date on which the consent is signed;
8. A statement that the consent is subject to revocation at any time except to the extent that the program or person which is to make the disclosure has already acted in reliance on it; and
9. The date, event or condition upon which the consent will expire if not revoked before.[55]

A use or disclosure *may not be made* if the consent has expired, is known to have been revoked, on its face substantially fails to conform with any of the requirements set forth above, or is known, or through a reasonable effort could

---

55 42 CFR § 2.31.

be known, to be materially false. Additionally, each disclosure or use of such health information must include the following written statement:

> This information has been disclosed to you from records protected by federal confidentiality rules (42 C.F.R. Part 2). The federal rules prohibit you from making any further disclosure of this information unless further disclosure is expressly permitted by the written consent of the person to whom it pertains or as otherwise permitted by 42 C.F.R. Part 2. A general authorization for the release of medical or other information is NOT sufficient for this purpose. The federal rules restrict any use of the information to criminally investigate or prosecute any alcohol or drug abuse patient.

A judge may authorize the disclosure or use of alcohol or drug abuse health information if the judge determines there is sufficient justification for the use or disclosure. The judge must determine that good cause exists and that the public interest and need for the use or disclosure outweigh the potential injury to the patient, the relationship between the patient and health care provider, and the treatment services.

B. HIV/AIDS

The diagnoses of human immunodeficiency virus (HIV) and acquired immunodeficiency syndrome (AIDS) have become major public policy issues because of their significant potential to adversely affect persons with such diagnoses. Many States have enacted laws that provide specific protections for these persons and their health information. These include requiring that health information that includes HIV status or AIDS as a diagnosis only be disclosed pursuant to an authorization that specifically identifies such information. It is recommended that this delineation be included in the Authorization required by the HIPAA Privacy Rule.

C. Mental Health

All States have specific laws governing mental health information, and there are also Federal laws relating to mental health information.[56] Recent legislation establishes an operative protection and advocacy system for patients with mental illness, including investigating incidents of abuse and neglect. States must have internal agencies to implement this Federal legislation, with these agencies having certain rights. These include:

---

56 The Protection and Advocacy for Mentally Ill Individuals Act of 1986, 42 U.S.C. § 10801 et seq.

1. Any individual who is a client of the system if such individual, or the legal guardian, conservator, or other legal representative of such individual, has authorized the system to have such access;

2. Any individual (including an individual who has died or whose whereabouts are unknown),

   a. who by reason of the mental or physical condition of such individual is unable to authorize the system to have such access;

   b. who does not have a legal guardian, conservator, or other legal representative, or for whom the legal guardian is the state; and

   c. with respect to whom a complaint has been received by the system or with respect to whom as a result of monitoring or other activities, either of which result from a complaint or other evidence, there is probable cause to believe that such individual has been subject to abuse or neglect;

3. Any individual with a mental illness, who has a legal guardian, conservator, or other legal representative, with respect to whom a complaint has been received by the system or with respect to whom there is probable cause to believe the health or safety of the individual is in serious and immediate jeopardy, whenever

   a. such representative has been contacted by such system upon receipt of the name and address of such representative;

   b. such system has offered assistance to such representative to resolve the situation; and

   c. such representative has failed or refused to act on behalf of the individual.

To the extent that there is a conflict between a State law and this Federal law, the Supremacy Clause of the Constitution is implicated and the Federal law will preempt the State statute under the following circumstances:

1. Congress can adopt express language setting forth preemption of the Federal law;

2. State law is preempted where Congress creates a scheme of Federal regulations so pervasive as to leave no room for supplementary State regulations; and

3. State law is preempted to the extent that it actually conflicts with Federal law.[57]

---

[57] *Oklahoma Disability Law Center, Inc. v. Dillon Family & Youth Services, Inc.*, 879 F. Supp. 1110 (N.D. Ok. 1995).

Under both this Federal law and many State laws, information about mental health patients may be withheld from disclosure to the patient if such disclosure would be detrimental to the patient's health.

D. Deceased Patients

A firm legal principle is that the privacy and confidentiality of health information survives a patient's death. However, many States do not identify who has the authority to access health information of a deceased patient. Certainly if the patient has a legal guardian or had a designated agent under a durable power of attorney for health care or similar document, such person is entitled to use and disclose the deceased patient's health information. Another alternative is to identify those persons entitled to bring a lawsuit as a result of the patient's death who may need access to the deceased patient's health information for purposes of such litigation. Some reasonable measures must be taken to prevent the unauthorized use or disclosure of a deceased person's health information.

In *Spearman v. Western Missouri Mental Health Center*[58], the parent of a patient who died after choking on a sandwich attempted to obtain copies of the health information of her son. Western Missouri Mental Health Center took the position that the patient's health information was deemed confidential by a Missouri statute and there wasn't any other statutory provision that permitted the release. The Court noted that Missouri law provided that health information of a patient could be disclosed to a legally authorized representative of the patient. As the appointed representative of her son's estate, the court held that the parent stood as the authorized legal representative.

SECTION 6-7: LIABILITY EXPOSURES

A. Defamation

An action for defamation arises when a verbal or written statement injures the reputation and good name of a patient. Statements of hatred, contempt, or ridicule, or that diminish esteem, respect, good will, or confidence in a patient can be defamatory. Even statements pertaining to insanity, poverty, rape, and drunkenness have been held to be defamatory.

If the communication is written, it is libel; oral defamation is slander. The elements essential for a successful defamation action are:

    1. Written or oral communication;

        a. Communication to a third party;

---

58 108 S.W.3d 801 (Mo. App. W.D. 2003).

    b. Causes injury to reputation or good name; and

    c. Communication pertains to a living person.

Truth is a defense in defamatory actions. Another defense is that the communication was made with the patient's consent.

Many State laws provide immunity for communications considered to be "absolutely privileged." These are statements otherwise actionable but are immune from defamation allegations because they were made to further some interest of social importance. Examples of absolute privileges are communications made in judicial and legislative proceedings, executive meetings, administrative proceedings, and political broadcasts.

A "qualified privilege" may be afforded if a communication is based on a proper motive and made with reasonable care to ascertain the truth. The communication must be made in the discharge of a public or private duty, whether legal or moral.

Certain slanderous statements are actionable as a matter of law without proof of any damage:

1. Crime involving moral turpitude or an infamous punishment, usually involving a major social disgrace;

2. Loathsome disease, such as venereal diseases;

3. Statements with reference to a matter of significance and importance to the person's business, trade, profession, or office; or

4. Unchastity, such as adultery, fornication, serious sexual misconduct, or deviant sexual behaviors.

Damages available in defamation actions include compensatory or actual damages, punitive damages, and nominal damages.

B. Invasion Of Privacy

An invasion of privacy occurs when conduct exceeds the limits of decency and offends a person of ordinary sensibilities. The four possible acts constituting invasion of privacy are:

1. Unreasonable intrusion upon the seclusion of another;

2. Public disclosure of private facts;

3. Publicity that places another in false light before the public; and

4. Appropriation of the name or likeness of another.

Authorization to disclosure of the private information is a complete defense.

C. Loss or Negligent Destruction of Health Information

The loss or destruction of health information can be extremely damaging to health care providers

In *DeLaughter v. Lawrence County Hospital*, the issue was whether the jury was entitled to be told why the original medical record was missing.[59] The evidence in this case was that the hospital refused to release the patient's medical record to her family without proper authorization. On the day of the patient's death, the Director of Nursing instructed the records custodian to lock up the patient's record so that the family could not get it. When the records custodian attempted to comply with the instructions, she discovered that the patient's medical record was missing. The record had last been seen two or three days prior to the patient's death, sitting in the physicians' box awaiting dictation. Upon discovery that the record was missing, the hospital set about reconstructing the file by gathering copies of items from the various medical departments within the hospital. However, even when reconstructed, the record was incomplete because it lacked the medical history, physical assessments, and the nursing progress notes.

The Mississippi Supreme Court held that the jury was entitled to hear that the hospital's original medical record was lost as that was a relevant fact. The burden was on the hospital to explain why the medical record was missing.

Several courts have held that there is a rebuttable presumption shifting the burden of persuasion to a health care provider who negligently alters or loses medical records relevant to a malpractice claim. This issue was thoroughly discussed by the Alaska Supreme Court in *Sweet v. Sisters of Providence in Washington.*[60]

Jacob Sweet allegedly sustained brain damage while a patient at Providence Hospital in Anchorage. His parents brought an action against Providence Hospital and several physicians claiming that their negligence caused Jacob's severe brain injury. The Sweets also alleged that Providence Hospital's inability to locate certain medical records precluded them from proving medical negligence and that they were entitled to recover based on a claim of intentional or negligent spoliation of evidence.

Jacob was born at Providence Hospital on January 16, 1988. Dr. Tulip examined him shortly after birth and found nothing abnormal about the infant's health. The next day Jacob was circumcised. The Sweets contend that they were never advised that they had any choice in deciding whether Jacob should be circumcised. Mrs. Sweet stated that she had not discussed circumcision with any physicians and a nurse presented her with the authorization. She signed the authorization because

---

59 601 So.2d 818 (Miss. 1992).

60 881 P.2d 304 (Alaska 1994).

she believed that all baby boys were circumcised and didn't know she had a choice in the matter. Neither the nurse nor any physicians had any independent recollection of talking with Mrs. Sweet about Jacob's circumcision.

Jacob was discharged from the hospital on January 18. One week later, the Sweets called Dr. Tulip because Jacob had become fussy and was vomiting. Jacob's circumcision site also appeared red and swollen.

Dr. Tulip met the Sweets in the Emergency Room at approximately 11:00 p.m. He examined Jacob and determined that he had a localized infection in his penis. Recognizing that infants are at high risk for developing potentially life-threatening systemic bacterial infections, Dr. Tulip admitted Jacob for IV antibiotic therapy.

There are numerous critical facts at issue regarding Jacob's condition and treatment between the time he was admitted and the time he was transferred to the NICU, approximately 26 hours later. Although a number of medical records exist that set forth some specifics regarding Jacob's care during this twenty-six hour period, missing records include Jacob's narrative nursing notes, a medication sheet, a graphic record, and a nursing care flow sheet. These notes have been called the "eyes and ears of the doctor." The Sweets claimed that the missing records precluded them from succeeding on their medical negligence claims, and that as a result they were entitled to a presumption of negligence.

The court found that two determinations needed to be made to judge the effect of the missing records. First, there must be a preliminary determination of the potential importance of the missing records before shifting the burden—whether the absence of the records sufficiently hinders the plaintiffs' ability to proceed. Second, the burden shifting will only occur if the essential medical records are missing through the negligence or fault of the hospital. Based on the facts in this case, there should be a rebuttable presumption that Providence Hospital was medically negligent in treating Jacob and that this negligence legally caused his injuries, absent a jury finding that the hospital's failure to maintain Jacob's records was excused. There January 26 nursing records contain material and substantial evidence of the conduct of Providence Hospital with respect to Jacob. The absence of this information clearly hinders the ability of the Sweets to proceed. It is also clear that Providence Hospital has the responsibility of preserving Jacob's medical records.

D. Breach of Fiduciary Duty

The common practice of health care providers and health information managers to mail requested health information in response to a subpoena to attend a deposition was the issue addressed by the Missouri Appellate Court in *Fierstein v.*

DePaul Health Center.[61] DePaul Health Center received a subpoena duces tecum to appear at a deposition with the medical records of Judy Fierstein. The subpoena was related to a lawsuit filed by Mrs. Fierstein's ex-husband, Dr. Fierstein, to modify his custodial rights of their children. Dr. Fierstein's attorney issued the subpoena duces tecum along with a letter indicating that the requested medical records could be mailed prior to the date of the deposition to avoid the medical records custodian having to appear at the deposition. DePaul's medical records custodian executed an affidavit and immediately mailed the requested medical records to Dr. Fierstein's attorney. It was undisputed that Mrs. Fierstein never gave DePaul her consent or authorization for the release of her medical records. Mrs. Fierstein filed a lawsuit against DePaul alleging that the release of her medical records violated the physician-patient privilege as well as fiduciary and ethical duties owed her by DePaul.

The law is clear that a physician has a fiduciary duty of confidentiality, and that hospital medical records are included under this privilege. "If a physician discloses any information, without first obtaining the patient's waiver, then the patient may maintain an action for damages in tort against the physician."[62] The court concluded that DePaul clearly released Mrs. Fierstein's medical records in violation of this subpoena, regardless of the letter from Dr. Fierstein's attorney. Thus, Mrs. Fierstein has alleged sufficient facts to support an actionable claim against DePaul Health Center.

Mrs. Fierstein proceeded to trial against DePaul for the wrongful release of her medical records. The jury returned verdicts in favor of her, awarding her $10,000 in actual damages and $375,000 in punitive damages. DePaul Health Center subsequently appealed.

DePaul asserted that the plaintiff failed to make a submissible case for punitive damages and she failed to prove DePaul's conduct was outrageous and/or motivated by evil intent or reckless indifference. DePaul claimed "Its release of the medical records was done in good faith and with the honest belief that its conduct was lawful."[63] Punitive damages are appropriate where the conduct of the defendant is outrageous because of reckless indifference to the rights of others. DePaul's medical records custodian testified that she telephoned the office of the attorney for Dr. Fierstein and talked to a male employee to confirm that Mrs. Fierstein's attorney had consented to the release of the records. The only man employed in that attorney's office testified he did not recall talking to the medical records custodian and that if he had spoken with her, he would not

---

61   *Fierstein v. DePaul Health Center*, 949 S.W.2d 90 (Mo. App. E.D. 1997), *affirmed*, 24 S.W.3d 220 (Mo. App. E.D. 2000).

62   949 S.W.2d at 92.

63   24 S.W.3d at 224.

have told her there was a consent to release the medical records. Because of the conflicting testimony, the jury was free to disbelieve the testimony of the DePaul's medical records custodian that she made a good faith attempt to verify the consent to release the medical records. Given the gravity of the information contained in the medical records, the jury was entitled to view the conduct as exhibiting a reckless indifference to the rights of Mrs. Fierstein to have her medical records remain private.

The admissibility of a patient's blood-alcohol test result was the issue addressed in *Harmon v. State*,[64] Derek Harmon drove a car into a concrete barrier. The police officer at the scene noticed that he had a strong odor of alcohol on his breath and swayed when standing. He also found two tumblers containing alcohol in his car. Mr. Harmon was taken to the hospital because he was injured. After learning that blood was being drawn from Mr. Harmon, the officer obtained a grand jury subpoena requesting Mr. Harmon's medical records from the hospital, including chemical or blood alcohol results. The medical records reflected that the blood alcohol content was 0.18.

Mr. Harmon contended that the State did not meet its burden to prove the reasonableness of the search and he had a statutory right to privacy under the HIPAA Privacy Rule. Because there is little societal interest in safeguarding the privacy of medical records when blood-alcohol tests are obtained by medical personnel after traffic accidents, courts have held that there is no legitimate expectation of privacy in such information. There is no Fourth Amendment reasonable expectation of privacy that protects blood test results of an injured motorist from being given to law enforcement officers pursuant to a grand jury subpoena. The court further noted that under the HIPAA Privacy Rule, it is permissible without the patient's permission to disclose medical records for law enforcement purposes and pursuant to a grand jury subpoena.

E. Nurse's Breach of Patient Confidentiality

A nurse who disclosed health information of numerous patients to an attorney to use in a lawsuit against the nurse's employer was found by the Kansas Supreme Court to have been legitimately discharged for breach of confidentiality.[65] Allison Goodman was terminated by Wesley Medical Center when it became aware that she had released names and treatment information for Wesley patients to attorney Brad Prochaska.

In May 2000, Wesley was a defendant in a lawsuit alleging negligence due to understaffing. Although Nurse Goodman had not been involved in the medical care of the involved patient, Mr. Prochaska contacted her after hear-

---

64 2003 WL 21665488 (Tx. App. 1st Dist. 2003).

65 *Goodman v. Wesley Medical Center, LLC*, 78 P.3d 817 (Kan. 2003).

ing she was willing to be a witness for him. Nurse Goodman agreed to be a witness and gave him documents from Wesley Medical Center that she contended would substantiate the claim of understaffing. When Nurse Goodman's supervisor asked her if she had provided the documents to Mr. Prochaska, she responded by stating that she "did nothing wrong." Nurse Goodman was then terminated for breaching Wesley Medical Center's policy concerning patient confidentiality.

Nurse Goodman alleged that in fact Wesley had terminated her in retaliation for reporting Wesley's alleged unsafe nursing practices. After thorough discussion of the retaliation claim, the court concluded the only evidence disputing Wesley's motive for terminating Nurse Goodman came from Nurse Goodman; there was no other evidence other than her own suspicions to back up her claim. Nurse Goodman argued that she did not breach confidentiality because when she provided the documents to Mr. Prochaska, since they were "communications between herself and Prochaska, her attorney," and as such were communications protected by the attorney/client privilege. The Court kindly noted that it was clear Nurse Goodman lacked an understanding of what the attorney/client privilege entails, and she failed to offer any legal authority for her arguments. Nurse Goodman then attempted to argue that Mr. Prochaska was "entitled to the information;" however, again Nurse Goodman failed to supply any legal authority to support such a proposition. In her last attempt to defend her actions, Nurse Goodman claimed there was no breach of confidentiality because no one saw the documents other than Mr. Prochaska. She was evidently unaware, or denying, the fact that the medical records and other documents she provided to Mr. Prochaska had been filed with the District Court, that Mr. Prochaska saw the documents when he was not involved in treating those patients, and there was absolutely no waiver of confidentiality or authority to share such documents with Mr. Prochaska.

F. Documentation: Deficiencies and Strategies

A heartwarming case for nurses was issued by the Louisiana Court of Appeals in 2003.[66] Lucille Reagan was a resident at the Glen Oak Retirement Home in June 1992. At that time, she was 79 years old and had Alzheimer's Disease, depression, cerebral atherosclerosis, senile dementia with delirium, and chronic mental syndrome. In July 1996, Mrs. Reagan was diagnosed with Stage 2 cancer and underwent a colon resection. Mrs. Reagan's daughters filed suit against the Glen Oak Retirement Home alleging: (1) failure to properly chart on Mrs. Reagan, including her bowel habits and constipation beginning in June 1995; (2) failing to effectively monitor Mrs. Reagan's medical records and properly coor-

---

[66] *Hinson v. The Glen Oak Retirement System*, 853 So.2d 726 (La. App. 2nd Cir. 2003).

dinate her care plan; (3) failing to effectively communicate with Mrs. Reagan's doctor; (4) failing to properly chart about Mrs. Reagan that resulted in a substantial delay in diagnosing her colon cancer; and (5) Mrs. Reagan lost a chance of survival by virtue of the delayed diagnoses of her condition.

At trial, there was evidence that nurses failed to properly chart, monitor, and address Mrs. Reagan's condition and to coordinate her care plan, and that these omissions lead to ineffective communication with Mrs. Reagan's physician. Linda McWatters, who was the Director of Nursing at the Glen, testified that to get a true picture of a resident's condition at any given moment, one can't simply look at the care plan and monthly nursing summaries; there are also nurses notes, forms, summaries from other disciplines such as pharmacy, dietary, and social services. Regarding the nursing flow sheets, certified nursing assistants are responsible for documenting activities of daily living, such as bowel movements. However, documentation of a bowel movement requires actual observation by the CNA.

There was further testimony that the State laws for nursing homes only required clinical records to contain sufficient information to identify the resident, provide a record of the resident's assessment, the plan of care, an explanation of services provided, progress notes, and the results of the preadmission screening. Laboratory services are only obtained when ordered by the resident's physician.

As Ms. McWatters testified, constipation is the most common problem nursing residents experience and is not in and of itself indicative of colon cancer. Warning signs for colon cancer usually include significant weight loss, significant change in eating habits, noticeable behavioral changes, significant changes in bowel habits, and rectal bleeding. In reviewing Mrs. Reagan's medical record, it was evident that her physician was seeing her on a regular basis and was fully cognizant of Mrs. Reagan's constipation. There was never a trend or pattern of constipation such that the nursing staff should have been alerted to the fact that Mrs. Reagan had colon cancer.

It wasn't until the end of June 1996 that Mrs. Reagan's medical record indicated she was sleeping more, becoming less active and involved, and was agitated. As a result of a fall, her physician ordered lab work which revealed anemia and caused him to order occult blood testing, which revealed blood in her stool. After a significant amount of expert testimony on both sides, the court concluded that although Mrs. Reagan's bowel movements were rather haphazardly charted by the nurses and other nursing home staff, there was no evidence of causal connection between the failure to document all of Mrs. Reagan's bowel activities and the delayed diagnosis of her colon cancer. Thus, the failure to discern the fact that Mrs. Reagan was suffering from colon cancer could not be laid upon the shoulders of the nurses and nursing staff of the Glen Oak Retirement Home.

In another Louisiana case, it was alleged that nurses were negligent in maintaining bed rails in place to prevent that patient from falling.[67] As is required in Louisiana, claims must be initially submitted to a Medical Review Panel. The Medical Review Panel found the evidence did not support the claim that Memorial Hospital failed to comply with the appropriate standard of care. The reasons submitted by the panel included:

> The evidence presented, in the form of hospital records and nurses notes (which were appropriate and thorough) strongly indicate that proper treatment was being rendered to the patient, and more specifically, that the hospital staff had been consistent in keeping the bedrails up to prevent injury to the patient. Literally every shift on the "Nursing Flow Records" from the date of admission on July 23, 1993 up to 30 minutes before the incident in question on the morning of July 26, 1993, and afterwards, indicate that the bedrails were checked and were up, either times 2 or times 4 position. Our opinion is based on the actual records presented for review as opposed to any post-incident recollections by the parties involved, although some concern arises from the fact that the relative of the patient who slept in the hospital room every night apparently was not following nurses instructions as to the patient's restraints even several days after the incident, according to the nurses notes of July 2, 1993.[68]

In addition to the comprehensive documentation, the plaintiff also failed to produce any expert testimony pertaining to the use of bedrails with patients such as Mrs. Thomas. The court concluded that there was not sufficient evidence establishing that the standard of care applicable to the nursing staff at Memorial Hospital with regard to appropriate use of bedrails was not met.

REFERENCES

AHIMA, *Practice Brief: Managing Health Information in Facility Mergers and Acquisitions* (1996).

AHIMA, *Practice Brief: Managing Health Information Relating to Infection with the Human Immunodeficiency Virus (HIV)* (1999).

AHIMA, *Practice Brief: Protecting Patient Information After A Facility Closure* (1999)

---

67 *Thomas v. Southwest Louisiana Hospital Ass'n*, 833 S.2d 548 (La. App. 3rd Cir. 2002).

68 *Id.* at 550.

AHIMA, *Practice Brief: Required Content For Authorizations to Disclose* (October 2002).

Amatayakul, M., Brandt, M. D., and Dennis, J. C., *Implementing the Minimums Necessary Standard/AHIMA Practice Brief)*, 73 Journal of AHIMA 96A (2002).

American Health Information Management Association, *Statement on the Privacy, Confidentiality, and Security of Health Records* (July 10, 2003), at http://library.ahima.org/.

American Hospital Association, Ad Hoc Committee on Hospital Closures, *Guidelines For Managing Hospital Closures* (1990).

American Medical Association and Health Care Financing Administration, *Documentation Guidelines for Evaluation and Management Services* (Nov. 1997).

At the Heart of HIPAA Privacy: Use and Disclosure for "Treatment", 2 Report on Patient Privacy 3 (Nov. 2002), at http://www.AISHealth.com.

Bishop, R. H., *The Final Patient Privacy Regulations Under the Health Insurance Portability and Accountability Act: Promoting Patient Privacy or Public Confusion?* 37 Georgia Law Review 723 (Winter 2003).

Case Law Development: Confident/Privacy, 27 Mental and Physical Disability Law Reporter 543 (July/August 2003).

Centers for Disease Control and Prevention, *HIPAA Privacy Rule and Public Health: Guidance From CDC and the U.S. Department of Health and Human Services,* 52 Morbidity and Mortality Weekly Report (April 11, 2003).

Doscher, M. and Davenport, C., *HIPAA's Final Security Rule,* HealthLeaders News (June 23, 2003), at http://www.healthleaders.com/news/print;php?contentid=46110.

Dougherty, M., *Accounting and Tracking Disclosures of Protected Health Information* (AHIMA Practice Brief), 72 Journal of AHIMA 72E (2001).

Duckett, G. M. and Burns, J., *Responding to Subpoenas For Medical Records In Compliance With HIPAA,* 39 Tennessee Bar Journal 18 (May 2003).

Glaser, J., *The Strategic Application of Information Technology in Healthcare Organizations* (2002).

Gradle, B. D., *National Accreditation Standards and HIPAA: A Comparative Chart,* 35 Journal of Health Law 577 (Fall 2002).

Hartin, T. A., *Balancing Federal and Wisconsin Medical Privacy Laws,* 76 Wisconsin Lawyer 10 (June 2003).

Health Information Compliance Insider, *A Plain-English Guide to HIPAA Privacy and Security Regulations,* Healthcare Information and Management Systems Society, at http://www.brownstone.com.

HIMSS/Phoenix Health Systems, *US Healthcare Industry Quarterly HIPAA Survey Results: Spring 2003,* at http://www.hipaadvisory.com/action/surveynew/Spring2003.htm.

Hjjort, B., *HIPAA Privacy and Security Training* (AHIMA Practice Brief), 73 Journal of AHIMA 60A (2002).

Hughes, G., *Defining The Designated Record Set* (AHIMA Practice Brief), 74 Journal of AHIMA 64A (2003).

Hughes, G., *Understanding the Minimum Necessary Standard* (AHIMA Practice Brief), 73 Journal of AHIMA 56A (2002).

Kreider, N. and Haselton, B., (editors), *The Systems Challenge: Getting the Clinical Information Support You Need To Improve Patient Care,* American Hospital Publishing, Inc. (1997).

Kumekawa, J. K., *Health Information Privacy Protection: Crisis or Common Sense?* 6 Online Journal of Issues in Nursing (September 30, 2001), at http://www.nursingworld.org/ojin/topic16/tpc16_2.htm.

Lyncheski, J. E., *The Impact of HIPAA On Employers*, Health Lawyers News, American Health Lawyers Association (December 2002).

Maneu, M., Whitten, P., and Allen, A., *E-Health Telehealth and Telemedicine* (2001).

Menenberg, S. R. *Standards of Care in Documentation of Psychiatric Nursing Care,* 9 Clinical Nurse Specialist 140 (1995).

Office of Civil Rights, *Standards For Privacy of Individually Indentifiable Health Information* (December 3, 2002).

Palmer, C., and Mickelson, L., *Falling Through the Cracks: The Unique Circumstances of HIV Disease Under Recent Americans With Disabilities Act Caselaw and Emerging Privacy Practices*, 21 Law and Inequality 219 (Summer 2003).

Practice Resource: *Sample Business Associate Addendum*, 36 Journal of Health Law 175 (Winter 2003).

Practice Resource: *Sample E-Mail Usage Policy for Healthcare Organizations*, 36 Journal of Health Law 365 (Spring 2003).

Ratner, S. B., *HIPAA's Preemption Provision: Doomed Cooperative Federation*, 35 Journal of Health Law 523 (Fall 2002).

Ryland, F., *Federal Health Privacy Comes to Maryland: What's the Big Deal?* 36 Maryland Bar Journal 26 (January/February 2003).

Taylor, C. O., and Marks, H. W., *Release of Medical Records: Current Status of Louisiana Law,* 51 Louisiana Bar Journal 18 (June/July 2003).

Top Type 1 Data Points to Lack of Documentation in Home Care and Hospice, 2 Briefings on JCAHO Home Health and Hospice (May 1999), at http://www.hin.com

U.S. Department of Health and Human Services, Website for HIPAA at http://www.hhs.gov/ocr/hipaa.

Yu, F. Y., *Medical Information Privacy Under HIPAA: A Practical Guide*, 32 Colorado Lawyer 11 (May 2003).

CHAPTER 7

Informed Consent

SECTION 7-1: PRINCIPLES AND APPLICABLE LAWS

A. Historical Basis of Doctrine

No longer are patients willing to accept on faith treatment decisions made by health care providers. Because public attitudes have shifted, the number of lawsuits alleging failure to obtain consent or lack of informed consent have significantly risen. In a study conducted on informed consent issues with endoscopists, 42% reported that in lawsuits brought against them, the informed consent process was an issue.[1]

Initially, physicians merely had to obtain the patient's agreement to undergo a proposed treatment. The physician had no responsibility to inform the patient about the proposed treatment, The risks or benefits, or any alternatives. Failure to obtain a patient's agreement constituted battery, the unauthorized touching of another.

In 1957, California required that information regarding the proposed treatment be provided to patients prior to obtaining consent.[2] This created the legal doctrine of "informed consent" as we know it today. Subsequent to this, the Supreme Court of Kansas became the first court to expressly hold a physician liable for negligence rather than battery based upon lack of informed consent.[3] "Failure to obtain informed consent" is malpractice.

The premises for requiring that information be provided to patients are:

---

1   Levine, E.G., et al., *Informed Consent: A Survey of Physician Outcomes and Practices.* Gastrointestinal Endoscopy 41 (1995): 448.

2   *Salgo v. Leland Stanford Jr. Univ. Bd. of Trustees*, 317 P.2d 170 (Cal. App. 1957).

3   *Natanson v. Kline*, 350 P.2d 1093 (Kan. 1960), *reh'g denied*, 354 P.2d 670 (Kan. 1960).

1. Patients are generally persons unlearned in the medical sciences and, therefore, except in rare cases, courts may safely assume the knowledge of the patient and physician are not in parity;

2. An adult who is competent has the right to exercise control over what medical treatments are personally rendered;

3. To be effective, a patient's consent to treatment must be an *informed* consent; and

4. The patient has an abject dependence upon and trust in the physician for the information that is relied upon during the decision-making process.[4]

B. Standards For Disclosure

There are two standards used to determine what constitutes negligence in informed consent actions. The professional standard, or old rule, defines the duty to disclose as limited to those disclosures that a reasonable health care provider would make under the same or similar circumstances. The landmark case establishing this standard states the general philosophy for the disclosure obligation:

> The duty of the physician to disclose, however, is limited to those disclosures which a reasonable medical practitioner would make under the same or similar circumstances. How the physician may best discharge his obligation to the patient in this difficult situation involves primarily a question of medical judgment. So long as the disclosure is sufficient to assure an informed consent, the physician's choice of plausible courses should not be called into question if it appears, all circumstances considered, that the physician was motivated only by the patient's best therapeutic interests and he proceeded as competent medical men would have done in a similar situation.[5]

Establishing this standard requires expert witness evidence. It has been challenged as being a paternalistic and authoritarian standard.

The alternative is the reasonable *patient* standard, also referred to as the materiality rule or new rule, which focuses on the informational needs of the average, reasonable patient. This standard requires disclosing all information relevant to a meaningful decisional process. An integral part of this obligation is the duty of *reasonable* disclosure.

---

4 *Cobbs v. Grant*, 502 P.2d 1, 9 (Cal. 1972).

5 *Natanson v. Kline*, 350 P.2d 1093, 1106 (Kan. 1960), *reh'g denied*, 354 P.2d 670 (Kan. 1960).

The argument that physicians should establish what is "reasonable" was analyzed by the California Supreme Court in *Cobbs:*

> Even if there can be said to be a medical community standard as to the disclosure requirement for any prescribed treatment, it appears so nebulous that doctors become, in effect, vested with virtual absolute discretion . . . Respect for the patient's right of self-determination on particular therapy demands a standard set by law for physicians rather than one which physicians may or may not impose upon themselves. Unlimited discretion in the physician is irreconcilable with the basic right of the patient to make the ultimate informed decision regarding the course of treatment to which he knowledgeably consents to be subjected.[6]

Establishing what is the reasonable patient standard is not an easy burden. It must be shown that:

1. A material risk existed that was unknown to the patient;
2. There was a failure to disclose that risk; and
3. The injury was a direct result of that risk.

In *Randall v. U.S.*[7], the patient, Jacqueline Randall, alleged that the physicians had not obtained her informed consent to perform a vaginal delivery; that they failed to warn her of the risks of delivering vaginally with genital warts, and failed to give her the option of a Cesarean section. As a result, her daughter, Kimberly, suffered from what is referred to Juvenile Onset Recurrent Respiratory Papillomatosis or Juvenile Laryngeal Papillomatosis (JLP).

Shortly after becoming pregnant in April, Ms. Randall had a pap smear test which came back positive. On July 31st, a colposcopic examination was performed to follow up the pap smear. The medical records for the July 31st examination reflected: "Few mildly dysplastic cells (CIN-I)." On October 3rd, a second colposcopic exam was performed. The results were noted as: "Marked inflammation present with a few koilocytes suggestive of condyloma." Condyloma is generally known as genital warts and is a subtype of Human Papilloma Virus (HPV); it is a sexually-transmitted disease. Ms. Randall testified that she did not learn the results of either colposcopic exam until *after* the birth of Kimberly.

Dr. Conetsco performed the October 3rd colposcopic exam of Ms. Randall. Although she observed white epithelium on Ms. Randall's cervix which could represent low grade dysplasia, HPV, or immature metaplasia, she didn't biopsy because Ms. Randall was pregnant.

---

6 *Cobb, supra,* at 10.

7 859 F. Supp. 22 (D.D.C. 1994).

In October 1986, small growths began to appear on Ms. Randall's genital area. One very large and painful growth caused her to end sexual intercourse with her husband. Although Ms. Randall testified she informed Dr. O'Connor about these growths, he denied this. Dr. O'Connor asserted that if Ms. Randall had complained of wart-like growths, he would have examined her and noted this exam on the OB records.

Dr. Collins testified that he examined Ms. Randall on November 24th but didn't include the genital area. The medical record of the visit states: "All well" and reflects no evidence of condyloma. Dr. Collins also contended that he would have examined Ms. Randall if she were complaining of lesions in her vagina.

Ms. Randall's next obstetrical visit was on December 29th at which time she saw Dr. Puckett. His medical notes didn't reflect genital condyloma or Ms. Randall's alleged complaints.

On December 31st, Ms. Randall experienced false labor. She testified Dr. Puckett examined her and asked what these "bumps" were. Dr. Puckett refuted asking such a question and testified he was competent to diagnose condyloma and would have noted its presence. He also testified that he would have ordered a syphilis test if growths appearing to be condyloma were present to ensure they were not secondary syphilis.

On January 1st, Ms. Randall had labor pains. She was examined by Dr. English; the medical records of this visit don't indicate the presence of condyloma.

Ms. Randall was next seen on January 16th by Dr. O'Connor. Dr. O'Connor testified that if Ms. Randall had complained of or if he had observed genital condyloma during the vaginal exam, he would have noted this in Ms. Randall's medical record.

Ms. Randall went into labor on January 18th. During the one and one-half days she was in labor, Drs. Puckett, LeBeau, Girerd, and Procter performed nine vaginal and cervical exams on Ms. Randall.

Dr. Procter subsequently diagnosed and treated Ms. Randall for condyloma based on an exam of the vulva on March 13th.

In determining whether consent is informed, the court noted that a particular peril must be divulged if it's "material to the patient's decision; all risks potentially affecting the decision must be unmasked."[8] "Materiality" is "when a reasonable person, in what the physician knows or should know to be the patient's position, would be likely to attach significance to the risk or cluster of risks in deciding whether or not to forego the proposed therapy."[9] Thus, the questions were:

---

8 *Id.* at 31.

9 *Id.*

1. Should the results of the June pap smear showing irregular cells have been disclosed to Ms. Randall?
2. Should Ms. Randall have been counseled to consider a cesarean versus a vaginal birth?
3. What would a reasonable person have decided?
4. Would it have made a difference if Kimberly had been born via cesarean section?

The court concluded that Ms. Randall was entitled to know the results of the June pap smear. "Due care may require a physician perceiving symptoms of a bodily abnormality to alert the patient to the condition."[10] In response to the other questions, the court concluded that Walter Reed, through its physicians, knew or should have known that Ms. Randall had HPV at the time of Kimberly's birth. The June pap smear and the October 3rd colposcopic exam were objective evidence of the onset and progression of the condyloma.

Walter Reed had information in its possession (Ms. Randall's OB and GYN Clinic records) that should have put all the physicians on notice as to Ms. Randall's condition. "The root cause of Walter Reed's difficulty in recording and disseminating Ms. Randall's condition to the several doctors attending her was the fact that the OB and GYN Clinics had separate facilities and kept separate records. The physicians in the OB Clinic did not have ready access to the colposcopy records, located in the GYN Clinic, indicating the development of HPV in Ms. Randall."[11]

The court concluded Ms. Randall was owed the duty of knowing the appreciable risks because of the need for treatment, the likelihood that injury will occur, and the seriousness of any injury that could follow. Dr. Kashima, an expert in otolaryngology, testified that he treated patients with JLP and knows the risk and causation associated between HPV and JLP better than any of the other expert witnesses who testified. Although not an obstetrician, he stated that a Cesarean section should have been performed to have prevented the risk of JLP being transmitted to Kimberly. Even the defendant's expert witness conceded that the connection between HVP and JLP was reported in the medical literature in 1986.

With informed consent cases, causation occurs when the disclosure of significant risks, incidental to treatment, would have resulted in a decision against the proposed approach. The court reasoned that a reasonably prudent person in Ms. Randall's position, having been made aware of the risk and severity of JLP in an infant, would have decided in favor of a Cesarean section. Thus, Ms.

---

10 *Id.*

11 *Id.*

Randall proved there was a duty owed to her by Walter Reed to have informed her as to the risks associated with a vaginal delivery, and therefore awarded medical costs in the amount of $78,720 for past expenses, $192,000 for future medical expenses, and $500,000 for the pain and suffering of Kimberly.

C. When Required

All States and the District of Columbia require informed consent either by statute or by case law. Consent is *always* required prior to any touching, which includes bathing, taking a blood pressure, administering a medication, or performing a surgical procedure. There is an implicit consent when a patient presents for medical treatment that allows "routine" procedures to be performed without specific informed consent. However, what constitutes a "routine" procedure is not defined. Generally, it is accepted that activities which are non-invasive and present very few risks fall into this category. However, a patient may revoke that implicit consent at any time, and any touching subsequent to that revoked consent constitutes a battery. If there is any doubt as to whether a procedure or treatment is routine, provide specific information to the patient so that informed consent is given, implicitly or directly.

Specific informed consent is required for procedures and treatments that are invasive or have potentially serious side effects or complications. The requirement for specific informed consent also has been extended to certain medications where the potential harm to patients is significant. The rationale is that patients need such information to decide whether to undertake treatment when there are inherent risks.

Examples of the types of procedures and treatments typically requiring specific informed consent include:

1. Major or minor surgery that involves entry into the body;
2. All procedures in which anesthesia is used;
3. Non-surgical procedures that involve more than a slight risk of harm or that may cause a change in body structure, such as:

   a. Medications;
   b. Chemotherapy;
   c. Hormone therapy;
   d. Myelograms;
   e. Intravenous pyelograms; and
   f. Arteriograms;

4. All forms of radiological therapy;
5. Electroconvulsive therapy;

6. Experimental procedures; and
7. Transfusions of blood or blood products.

D. Exceptions

Emergency

In emergencies, consent generally is implied by law or as a matter of public policy. Health care providers are deemed to be acting reasonably by presuming that the patient would authorize treatment if capacity to consent was present. "Emergencies" are broadly interpreted to extend to situations in which immediate treatment is necessary to prevent jeopardy of life, health, or limb, disfigurement, or impairment of faculties. In essence, an emergency exists where inaction might result in greater harm to the patient. Document the nature of the emergency and why consent cannot be obtained.

Therapeutic Privilege

The therapeutic privilege allows the withholding of information from a patient where it is believed that more harm will result by disclosing that information. To defend an assertion of therapeutic privilege, there must be strong evidence that the truth will create a greater harm than the lie. Recognize that withholding information may interfere with the patient's ability to give informed consent.

Waiver

A patient's right to consent may be personally waived. A patient may choose not to receive any information because of inability to deal with the stress-producing nature of that information. Legally, this is permissible and allows the health care provider to proceed as determined to be in the best interest of the patient. However, such waiver should be documented and perhaps even executed as an authorization for the health care provider to proceed on behalf of the patient.

Prior Knowledge

If a patient has knowledge about the proposed procedure or treatment because of previous personal experiences, or because the elements constituting informed consent are within common knowledge, providing information is not necessary prior to obtaining informed consent. However, there should be documentation reflecting how the patient is knowledgeable. Also, the best approach is to verify that the patient has the necessary information to make an informed decision and document that verification.

E. Capacity To Consent

Before a patient can consent, it must be determined that the patient has the *capacity* to consent to that procedure or treatment, an essential element for a valid consent. There is a distinction between "incapacity" and "incompetency" in determining whether a patient can consent.

Incompetency reflects one's ability to transact business or to execute binding documents. Incompetency is a legal judgment rendered by a court after hearing evidence.

Incapacity is determined based on the patient's functional ability to understand the nature of the medical condition; the risks of treatment and non-treatment; the risks and benefits of the particular proposed treatment; and the available alternatives. Accordingly, a patient has capacity if:

1. Understands information relative to that decision;
2. Can deliberate regarding the available choices, considering the patient's own values and goals; and
3. Able to communicate a decision, verbally or non-verbally.

While there is a presumption of decisional capacity, be attentive to clues of decisional incapacity. There are no fixed standards for determining decisional incapacity; it's beneficial to have determinations made as a collaborative effort by the most informed and involved health care providers. Re-evaluate the determination if any changes occur in the patient's condition.

There is no formalized definition as to the degree of certainty required to establish incapacity. Because the determination of incapacity is being made by non-legal professionals in a non-legal setting, the process is best facilitated by a medical approach rather than a legal approach. While an opinion "to a reasonable degree of medical certainty" is often used, that requires a certain level of legal determination. If the matter is brought before a court for review, it is likely that incapacity must be manifested by "clear and convincing evidence."

Capacity is evaluated on a sliding standard based upon the intensity and complexity of the treatment decision. As the risks of the decision increase, the standard for capacity becomes more stringent. Decisional capacity should be task specific—the patient may have the ability to make some decisions but not others.

Merely because a patient's preference is for action different from what the average person would choose isn't evidence of incapacity. Is it consistent with the known values of the patient? Document how the level of capacity was evaluated; this provides justification for the determination and how it was made. It also provides important information as to how frequently capacity needs to be reevaluated or how it may change in the future.

F. Authority To Consent

The person must have the *authority* to consent to the treatment. If the patient is an adult, a person who is age 18 years or older, the patient has the legal authority to consent to any personal treatment. This includes the right to *refuse* any treatment. If the patient lacks decisional capacity, who may consent for that patient will depend upon State law. For a patient who has been declared incompetent and a guardian appointed with the authority to make health care treatment decisions, the guardian then has the authority to consent. Some States limit the scope of decisions a guardian can make for an incompetent patient.

Many States have enacted legislation that allows a person to designate another individual to make health care treatment decisions when the patient lacks decisional capacity. This agency automatically becomes effective, allowing the agent to make health care treatment decisions.

Some States have enacted legislation designating family members as authorized to consent for the patient. Consent from family members of patients has been traditionally accepted even though they have no legal authority. Accepting such consent creates legal risks, although the alternative of forcing a family member to seek guardianship may not be in the patient's best interest. How to handle situations where no one has legal authority to consent, the patient lacks decisional capacity, and there aren't patient oral or written advance directories must be carefully examined to determine the best way, legally and ethically, to handle them.

An example where accepting consent from a family member who lacked authority to consent created a cause of action is reflected in *Mahurin v. St. Luke's Hospital of Kansas City.*[12] St. Luke's Hospital sued Mark and Denise Mahurin for the balance due on an unpaid hospital bill. The Mahurins counterclaimed for medical malpractice joining Dr. Spradlin and Dr. Hedegaard, alleging that each had committed medical malpractice in performing the tubal ligation on Mrs. Mahurin.

On October 21, 1985, Mrs. Mahurin was admitted to St. Luke's Hospital for childbirth. The baby was delivered by a Cesarean section. After the Cesarean section was performed consent was obtained from Mr. Mahurin to perform a bilateral tubal ligation on Mrs. Mahurin rendering her sterile. Mrs. Mahurin stated in an affidavit that she did not at any time request, authorize, or consent to a bilateral tubal ligation and that she was not advised during post-operative care that a tubal ligation had been performed.

An operation performed without a patient's consent is a battery or trespass. Consent to a given operation does not constitute consent for any other operation

---

12 809 S.W.2d 418 (Mo. App. 1991).

when there is no evidence that a necessity arose during the authorized opera-tion.[13] As the court noted: "There is no agency between a husband and wife merely because of the marital relationship and neither is empowered to act as agent for the other simply because they are married."[14] Thus, Mr. Mahurin's con-sent was not binding upon his wife since he had no authority to consent to the non-essential tubal ligation. The court concluded that Mrs. Mahurin is entitled to proceed with her claim against defendants for medical malpractice arising out of the unauthorized tubal ligation.

When the patient is a minor, consent for health care treatment must be obtained from a parent or legal guardian, or other person who is so authorized by law to consent in the absence of the parent or guardian.

States recognize some concept of "emancipated" minor, such as minors who are married, parents, or living independently of parental support, and per-mit emancipated minors to make personal health care decisions. Most States also have laws allowing minors to consent for specific types of treatment, such as drug and alcohol abuse, sexually transmitted diseases, pregnancy, contracep-tives, and abortion. The minor's right to consent to abortion was established by the United States Supreme Court in *Planned Parenthood of Central Missouri v. Danforth.*[15] However, States may place conditions on that right, although many of those have successfully been challenged for being unreasonable.

The need to obtain a valid consent to treat a minor is based on two separate legal reasons:

1. Liability for battery if there is no valid consent; and
2. Inability to obtain compensation for services if the consent is not given by someone with legal authority to make a binding contract for those services.

Document how the age was verified. How a court would view a misrepre-sentation of age by a minor is undetermined as there aren't any reported cases. However, in contract cases some courts have held that the minor's true age must be ascertained or suffer the consequences that the minor can disaffirm the con-tract, while others have ruled that minors cannot avoid a contract that has been procured by deceit. It is well advised to ask for proof of age before rendering care, especially for nonessential treatment.

Courts have addressed whether consent by a minor can be legally effective. In Illinois, a petition for neglect was filed against a 17-year-old girl's mother based on the mother's acquiescence to the daughter's decision to refuse, on reli-

---

13 *Id.* at 422.

14 *Id.*

15 428 U.S. 52 (1976).

gious grounds, blood transfusions that were necessary to prevent her from dying of leukemia. In *re E.G.*[16], E.G. was diagnosed with acute non-lymphatic leukemia. When E.G. and her mother, Rosie Denton, were informed that treatment of the disease involves blood transfusions, they refused to consent to them on the basis of their religious beliefs. As Jehovah's Witnesses, both E.G. and her mother desired to observe their religion's prohibitions against the "eating" of blood. Mrs. Denton authorized all other treatment for E.G.

As a result of the refusal to consent to blood transfusions, the State filed a neglect petition. Dr. Yachnin testified that without blood transfusions, E.G. would likely die within a month. He also testified that the transfusions, along with chemotherapy, achieve remission of the disease in about 80% of all patients so afflicted. However, the long-term prognosis was not optimistic, as a survival rate for patients such as E.G. was 20% to 25%. In Dr. Yachnin's opinion, E.G. was competent to understand the consequences of accepting or rejecting treatment and he was impressed with her maturity and the sincerity of her religious beliefs. Dr. Yachnin's observations regarding E.G.'s competency were also corroborated by the testimony of Jane McAtee, the Associate General Counsel for the University of Chicago Hospital.

When further hearings were held on the matter in April, E.G. testified that the decision to refuse blood transfusions was her own and that she fully understood the nature of her disease and the consequences of her decision. She indicated that her decision was not based on any wish to die but was grounded on her religious convictions. E.G. testified that when she had been forced to accept blood transfusions because of a prior court decision, she asked to be sedated prior to the administration of the blood because "it seems as if everything that I want or believe in is just being disregarded."

Several other witnesses gave their opinions about the sincerity of E.G.'s religious beliefs and her maturity to be able to make treatment decisions. Dr. Littner, a psychiatrist who has special expertise in evaluating the maturity and competency of minors, testified that based on his interviews with E.G., she had the maturity level of an 18 to 21-year old. In his opinion, E.G. had the competency to make an informed decision to refuse the blood transfusions, even if this choice was fatal.

The court noted that although the age of majority in Illinois is 18, "that age is not an impenetrable barrier that magically precludes a minor from possessing and exercising certain rights normally associated with adulthood."[17] As the court pointed out, there were many other Illinois laws that granted minors the legal authority to consent to medical treatment in certain situations: a minor 12 years

---

16 549 N.E.2d 322 (Ill. 1989).

17 *Id.* at 325.

or older could seek medical attention for a venereal disease or alcohol or drug abuse; a minor who is married or pregnant may validly consent to treatment; a minor 16 years or older may be declared emancipated under the Illinois Emancipation of Mature Minors Act and thereby control personal health care decisions. The court concluded that "the legislature did not intend that there be an absolute 18-year-old age barrier prohibiting minors from consenting to medical treatment."[18]

The court also took notice of several decisions of the United States Supreme Court that had adopted a mature minor doctrine, such as allowing women under the age of majority to undergo abortions without parental consent, and holding that children enjoy the protection of other constitutional rights, including the right to privacy, freedom from unreasonable searches and seizures, and procedural due process.

The court concluded that:

> [N]o bright line age restriction of 18 is tenable in restricting the rights of mature minors, whether the rights be based on constitutional or other grounds. Accordingly, we hold that in addition to these constitutionally based rights expressly delineated by the Supreme Court, mature minors may possess and exercise rights regarding medical care that are rooted in this State's common law."[19]

The issue of whether a 17-year-old minor had the capacity to consent was addressed by the Tennessee Supreme Court in Cardwell v. Bechtol.[20] Sandra Cardwell was 17 years old and suffered from persistent but intermittent back pain. At her own initiative, she decided to see Dr. Bechtol, an osteopath who had treated her father's back condition on several occasions in the past. Ms. Cardwell had not told her parents that she was seeing Dr. Bechtol.

Dr. Bechtol has been blind most of his life so he limits his practice to manipulative treatments to adjust or realign the skeletal system. He conducts a solo practice with the assistance of his wife and daughter, who maintain his records. He was alone in his office when Ms. Cardwell came to see him. She told Dr. Bechtol her name and that her father had been one of his patients. Ms. Cardwell also informed him of her symptoms and of the diagnoses of the orthopaedic specialists, that being that she had symptoms consistent with a herniated disc. Dr. Bechtol concluded, after examining Ms. Cardwell, that a herniated disc was not her problem and treated her with manipulations involving her neck, spine, and legs for a subluxation of the spine and bilateral sacroiliac slip.

18 *Id.* at 326.
19 *Id.* at 326.
20 724 S.W.2d 739 (Tenn. 1987).

The treatment lasted for about 15 minutes, after which Dr. Bechtol asked Ms. Cardwell to return several times during the next few weeks for further manipulations. Ms. Cardwell wrote her name, age, and address on a card Dr. Bechtol supplied her and then paid his fee of $25 with one of her father's blank, signed checks, which had been given to her to be used when she needed money.

After Ms. Cardwell left Dr. Bechtol's office, she experienced a tingling and numbing sensation in her legs. She went home and laid down to take a nap. She was awakened by severe pain about an hour later. The pain was such that she had difficulty walking but she was obligated to pick her mother up from work. Ms. Cardwell found that she had difficulty driving and when she reached her mother's place of employment her pain had become very intense. By the time she and her mother arrived at home, Ms. Cardwell was no longer able to walk by herself. She was taken to the Emergency Department at a hospital and was subsequently admitted. During the next few days, she underwent diagnostic testing which confirmed that she had a herniated disc. A laminectomy was performed. Although Ms. Cardwell's condition has improved gradually since her surgery, she had not yet regained normal bowel control, or complete sensation in her buttocks and one of her legs.

The allegations against Dr. Bechtol included medical malpractice and battery for failing to obtain the consent of Ms. Cardwell's parents. On the date of Ms. Cardwell's treatment by Dr. Bechtol, she was 17 years, 7 months of age, a senior in high school with good grades, and was planning to attend college. Testimony consistently characterized Ms. Cardwell as a mature young woman who acted somewhat older than her age. It was noted that on the day Ms. Cardwell went to see Dr. Bechtol, she had taken her mother's car so that she could also see the family physician about a sore throat. She had left school early and with her parents' permission had gone to this doctor's office alone, where she was examined and treated by the doctor who had not obtained parental consent.

In its discussion, the court acknowledged that minors achieve varying degrees of maturity and responsibility, thus reflecting capacity, and that this had been recognized as part of the common law for well over a century. "The rule of capacity has sometimes been known as the Rule of Sevens: under the age of seven, no capacity; between seven and fourteen, a rebuttable presumption of no capacity; between fourteen and twenty-one, a rebuttable presumption of capacity."[21] The court pointed out that this rule of capacity of minors had been applied in criminal cases and in determining the competency of minors to testify as witnesses.

---

21 *Id.* at 745.

The issue here is whether Ms. Cardwell had the capacity to consent to the treatment administered by Dr. Bechtol. Although plaintiffs contend that Ms. Cardwell failed to consent, the court disagreed:

> A person may, however, consent by conduct. By presenting herself to Defendant (Dr. Bechtol) for examination and treatment and then by submitting to treatment without protest or resistance, Defendant could reasonable conclude that he had Ms. Cardwell's consent to the treatment. "Consent is regarded as present, also, when one manifests a willingness that the defendant engage in conduct and the defendant acts in response to such a manifestation."[22]

The court emphasized that Ms. Cardwell was intelligent and capable for her age; the treatment was of a minor nature; Ms. Cardwell remained conscious throughout the treatment and was fully aware of what was being done; and Ms. Cardwell raised no objection to the procedure. The court concluded:

> Whether a minor has the capacity to consent to medical treatment depends upon the age, ability, experience, education, training, and degree of maturity or judgment obtained by the minor, as well as upon the conduct and demeanor of the minor at the time of the incident involved. Moreover, the totality of the circumstances, the nature of the treatment and its risks or probable consequences, and the minor's ability to appreciate the risks and consequences are to be considered. Guided by the presumptions in the Rule of Sevens, these are questions of fact for the jury to decide.[23]

From Ms. Cardwell's conduct in Dr. Bechtol's office and by her own testimony, the jury could conclude that Ms. Cardwell consented to the treatment. The court therefore upheld the jury's finding that Ms. Cardwell had the ability, maturity, experience, education, and judgment at her 17 years, 7 months of age to consent knowingly to medical treatment.

SECTION 7-2: PROCESS FOR INFORMED CONSENT

Obtaining an informed decision is a two-step process: (1) providing the information to the patient so that an informed decision can be made; and (2) obtaining consent. Each step has different requirements and, consequently, different responsibilities. The same person may be responsible for both steps or different people may assume accountability for each step.

---

22 *Id.* at 746.

23 *Id.* at 748.

A. Duty to Inform

The duty to inform the patient has repeatedly been held to belong to the person performing the procedure or treatment or the person ordering it. That is usually a physician. However, a nurse may act as the physician's agent in providing information to a patient.

In *Bulman v. Myers*, the patient questioned whether informed consent was obtained because information was provided by a nurse assistant and not by the operating surgeon.[24] Miriam Bulman was under the care of the defendant dentist, Dr. Myers. Ms. Bulman was admitted to the hospital for surgical removal of her maxillary and mandibular left and right third molars. Following surgery, Ms. Bulman suffered a marked loss of taste, temperature, and pain sensations in her tongue, and a slurring of speech. She alleged that the surgery was performed without her informed consent.

At trial, Ms. Bulman requested that the judge give the following instruction to the jury: "A patient cannot formulate a valid, informed consent to a surgical procedure when disclosures of the risks of surgery are made by a nurse assistant and not by the operating surgeon." Ms. Bulman testified that any information that she received concerning possible complications came only from the nurse assistant, who happened to also be Dr. Myers' wife. Mrs. Myers testified in detail as to the substance of the treatment information that she communicated to Ms. Bulman to enable her to make an informed decision.

The court rejected Ms. Bulman's assertion that only the physician can effectively relate the information necessary for an informed consent. The issue is the adequacy of the information given to Ms. Bulman, not the professional status of the person providing the information. Was there disclosure of all those facts, risks, and alternatives that a reasonable person in the situation would deem significant in making a decision to undergo the recommended treatment? The sufficiency of the information upon which the patient's consent is obtained is an issue for the jury. The court therefore affirmed the jury's verdict in favor of Dr. Myers.

In *Kus v. Sherman Hospital*, Richard Kus brought an action against Sherman Hospital, Dr. Vancil, and the manufacturers of the intraocular lenses that were implanted.[25] Mr. Kus settled with Dr. Vancil and the manufacturers prior to trial. Mr. Kus alleged that the Hospital committed a battery upon him and was negligent for failing to obtain informed consent.

Ms. Kus' vision began to deteriorate and he saw Dr. Vancil in January 1985. Dr. Vancil recommended cataract surgery and a lens implant which he alleged-

---

24 467 A.2d 1353 (Pa. Super. 1983).

25 644 N.E.2d 1214 (Ill. App. 1995).

ly told Mr. Kus were "quite safe." Mr. Kus testified that Dr. Vancil never told him that the lens Dr. Vancil intended to implant was under investigation for its safety and effectiveness. Dr. Vancil gave Mr. Kus a booklet that described intraocular lens implant surgery as a "tried and true method" of vision correction after cataract surgery. Prior to surgery, in Dr. Vancil's office, Mr. Kus was presented with a consent form, which Mr. Kus read and signed. Eye surgery proceeded on July 15, 1985, during which time Dr. Vancil implanted an intraocular lens into Mr. Kus' left eye.

Subsequently, Mr. Kus' vision deteriorated in his right eye and Dr. Vancil again recommended the implantation of an intraocular lens. Surgery on the right eye occurred on January 15, 1986, with allegedly no consent form in Mr. Kus' Hospital chart. Mr. Kus claimed he signed the consent form two to ten days after the surgery, and the form then appeared in his Hospital chart.

Prior to the implantations of the intraocular lenses into Mr. Kus, the Hospital IRB, which is charged with the responsibility to review and monitor all investigational studies, reviewed and approved the study for intraocular lenses. As part of its approval, the IRB approved a specific consent form to be used for patients undergoing intraocular lenses implantation. This consent form included a paragraph on "clinical investigation" to inform patients that the lens was under investigation for its safety and efficacy. A receptionist for Dr. Vancil testified that the consent forms in his office were missing the section on "clinical investigation;" Dr. Vancil had directed the office staff to remove that language from the consent form because "he didn't want it on there." This removal was done for all of Dr. Vancil's 43 patients who underwent intraocular lens surgery at Sherman Hospital.

Part of the IRB's responsibilities, as set forth in Federal regulations, is to "assure that the rights of human subjects are properly protected, that legally effective informed consent is obtained, and that the method of obtaining consent properly informs the human subject of the significant aspects of the study. . . ."[26] This requires that each subject be provided with this information: "A statement that the study involves research, an explanation of the purposes of the research and the expected duration of the subject's participation, a description of the procedures to be followed, and identification of any procedures which are experimental."[27] The patient's informed consent also must be on a form that has been approved by the IRB.

The court acknowledged that Sherman Hospital generally has no duty to obtain informed consent from the patient.[28] The rationale underlying this rule is that the physician has the "technical knowledge and training necessary to advise

---

26 *Id.* at 1218.

27 *Id.* at 1218.

28 *Id.* at 1220.

each patient of the risks," and that "the hospital does not know the patient's medical history, nor the details of the particular surgery to be performed."[29]

But the court found that the hospital was a participating institution in the study, and was charged with assuring that "legally effective informed consent" was obtained prior to the experimental surgery.[30] As a participating institution, Sherman Hospital is required to conduct "continuing review of research" under the Federal regulations, which includes the duty to review the informed consent process.[31] Sherman Hospital thus had the minimal duty of verifying that the consent form approved by its IRB was being used by Dr. Vancil.

Nurses may be required to verify that consent has been obtained prior to a procedure or treatment. If the nurse fails to make that verification, both the nurse and hospital could be negligent. Liability can also result if a hospital or nurse knows or should know of a physician's repeated failure to obtain informed consent or it becomes aware that consent has not been obtained.[32]

The information provided to the patient for an informed decision must be in writing or documented and include:

1. What information was told to the patient;
2. Whether anyone else was present during that discussion;
3. That an opportunity was given to the patient to ask questions;
4. The indication of understanding by the patient;
5. The amount of time spent discussing the proposed treatment or procedure with the patient;
6. Whether any materials were used in providing the information such as videos, anatomy drawings, or reading materials; and
7. Whether further discussions with the patient is warranted before a decision is made.

This documentation is critical when defending a malpractice action for lack of informed consent or failure to obtain consent when the patient denies that certain information was provided. It further provides the reasonable belief that the patient has been informed as needed by the nurse prior to witnessing a consent.

B. Elements

The five elements for a patient to make informed decisions include:

---

29 *Id.*

30 *Id.* at 1221.

31 *Id.*

32 *Krane v. Saint Anthony Hospital Systems*, 738 P.2d 75 (Colo. App. 1987).

1. The nature and purpose of the proposed procedure or treatment;
2. The expected outcome and the likelihood of success;
3. The material risks and frequency of their occurrence;
4. The alternatives and supporting information regarding those alternatives; and
5. The effect of no treatment or procedure, including the effect on the prognosis and the material risks associated with no treatment.

The amount of information given to the patient depends upon that patient's level of education, understanding, and interest. The information provided must be sufficient to allow that patient to be knowledgeable about what is being proposed, within the patient's personal level of understanding.

To evaluate the benefits of the proposed treatment or procedure, the patient needs to be told what is the likelihood of success and the expected outcome. This needs to be a realistic assessment based upon general statistics and the provider's personal clinical experience with that treatment.

The most common allegation is the failure to disclose material risks. Whether a risk is "material" is determined on a case-by-case basis. Courts have not defined materiality either in view of the frequency or severity of the risk, although those are significant factors. Materiality may be determined because of the effect on physical appearance or sexual or reproductive functioning.

Patients must be told of any *reasonable* alternatives and the supporting information about each of those alternatives. The choice of alternatives may involve value judgments as well as consideration of social, economical, and personal factors. Even though all alternatives may not accomplish the same outcome, they need to be explained as they may involve different levels of risks.

Finally, tell the patient what is likely to occur if *no* treatment or procedure is undertaken. This includes the prognosis for the patient as well as any risks inherent in refusing a treatment or procedure.

C. Obtaining Consent

Consent may be verbal or written, as may be required by Federal or State law, or by a facility policy. A *signed* consent form is not inherently evidence that consent is informed, unless State law so provides. The patient can still allege consent was not informed, although it will preclude an allegation of battery.

When witnessing consent, the witness is attesting to:

1. The authenticity of the signature on a consent form;
2. The patient has decisional capacity for that treatment decision;
3. The person is authorized to personally consent or consent for the patient;

4. Consent is being given freely, voluntarily, and without coercion; and

5. There is a reasonable belief that the patient has been informed so an informed decision can be made.

The authenticity of the signature means that the signature is that of the person signing and is not being forged.

The patient's decisional capacity is determined at the time the consent is being obtained. It is based upon an assessment of the patient's ability to make that health care decision, and to communicate that decision.

Verify that the person is authorized to personally consent or to consent for the patient, as discussed above.

Consent by a patient must be given freely and because that is the *patient's* choice, not because the physician or family members prefer that course of treatment. This is of special concern with elderly patients who may be more easily subjected to and influenced by these pressures.

Finally, the witness shall have a reasonable belief that the patient has been provided the essential information so that an informed decision is being made. This does not require that the witness must be present while information is discussed with the patient; at a minimum the witness verifies there was a discussion, the patient can communicate a basic understanding of what is being consented to, and the witness asks the patient if any further questions or clarifications need addressing before a decision can be made.

SECTION 7-3: MENTAL HEALTH PATIENTS

The right to consent to treatment is not automatically abrogated for mentally ill patients. Institutionalization, whether voluntary or involuntary, does not deny a patient the right to make personal treatment decisions. Commitment arises because it is believed that a patient could cause personal harm or endanger another person. Whether a patient has the mental ability to make a decision regarding personal health care treatment is an entirely separate and distinct issue.

This right to consent includes whether psychotropic medications can be administered. Courts have uniformly held that absent judicial authorization, forcible administration of psychotropic drugs is limited to either:

1. Emergencies in which the patient poses an imminent threat of personal harm or harm to others and there is no alternate less intrusive method available than forced medication; or

2. The medication is required to prevent an immediate, substantial, and irreversible deterioration of a patient's mental illness.

Remember, the first step in the consent process: does the patient have *capacity* to make an informed judgment? Consent given by a patient who lacked capacity was a significant issue in this case.[33] Darrell Burch brought an action against eleven physicians, administrators, and staff members at Florida State Hospital under 42 U.S.C. § 1983 which reads: "Every person who, under color of any statute, ordinance, regulation, custom, or usage, of any State . . . subjects, or causes to be subjected, any citizen of the United States, to the deprivation of any rights, privileges, or immunities secured by the Constitution and laws, shall be liable to the party injured in an action at law . . ." Mr. Burch alleged that defendants deprived him of his liberty, without due process of law, by admitting him to Florida State Hospital (FSH) as a voluntary mental patient when he was incompetent to give informed consent to his admission.

On December 7, 1981, Mr. Burch was found wandering along a Florida highway, appearing to be hurt and disoriented. He was taken to Apalachee Community Mental Health Services. The evaluation form stated that, upon his arrival at ACMHS, Mr. Burch was hallucinating, confused, and psychotic, and believed he was "in heaven." His face and chest were bruised and bloody, suggesting that he had fallen or had been attacked. Mr. Burch was asked to sign forms giving his consent to admission and treatment, which he did. He remained at ACMHS for three days, during which time the facility's staff diagnosed his condition as paranoid schizophrenia and gave him psychotropic medications.

On December Dr. Zinermon wrote a progress note indicating that Mr. Burch was "refusing to cooperate," "would not answer questions," "appears distressed and confused," and "related that medication has been helpful." Mr. Burch was then transferred to Florida State Hospital and signed forms requesting admission and authorizing treatment at FSH. One form, "Request for Voluntary Admission," recited that the patient requests admission for "observation, diagnosis, care and treatment of (my) mental condition" and that the patient, if admitted, agrees to accept such treatment a may be prescribed by members of the medical and psychiatric staff in accordance with the provisions of expressed and informed consent." Two of the defendants signed this form as witnesses. A nursing assessment form dated December 11 stated that Mr. Burch was confused and unable to state the reason for his hospitalization and still believed that "this is heaven."

On December 23rd, Mr. Burch signed another form entitled "Authorization for Treatment." This form stated that he authorized "the professional staff of (FSH) to administer treatment except electroconvulsive treatment"; that he had been informed of "the purpose of treatment; common side effects thereof; alternative treatment modalities; approximate length of care"; of his power to revoke

---

33 *Zinermon v. Burch*, 494 U.S. 113, 108 L. Ed. 2d 100, 110 S. Ct. 975 (1990).

consent to treatment; and that he had read and fully understood the authorization. Defendant Dr. Zinermon, also a staff physician at FSH, signed the form as the witness.

On December 29th, Dr. Zinermon documented that on admission Mr. Burch's condition was "disoriented, semi-mute, confused and bizarre in appearance and thought, not cooperative to the initial interview, and extremely psychotic, appeared to be paranoid and hallucinating." She also recorded that Mr. Burch remained disoriented, delusional, and psychotic. Mr. Burch remained at FSH until May 7, 1982, five months after his initial admission to ACMHS. During that time, no hearing was held regarding his hospitalization and treatment.

After his release, Mr. Burch complained that he had been admitted inappropriately to FHS and did not remember signing a voluntary admission form. In Mr. Burch's complaint, he alleged as follows:

> Defendants, and each of them, knew or should have known that Plaintiff was incapable of voluntary, knowing, understanding and informed consent to admission and treatment at FSH . . . Nonetheless, Defendants, and each of them, seized Plaintiff and against Plaintiff's will confined and imprisoned him and subjected him to involuntary commitment and treatment for the period from December 10, 1981, to May 10, 1982. For said period of 149 days, Plaintiff was without the benefit of counsel and no hearing of any sort was held at which he could have challenged his involuntary admission and treatment at FSH.
>
> . . .
>
> Defendants, and each of them, deprived Plaintiff of his liberty without due process of law in contravention of the Fourteenth Amendment to the United States Constitution. Defendants acted with willful, wanton and reckless disregard of and indifference to Plaintiff's Constitutionally guaranteed right to due process of law."

Under Florida's law, a short term emergency (involuntary) admission is appropriate if it is believed that a person is mentally ill, likely to injure himself or others or is in need of care or treatment, and lacks sufficient capacity to make a responsible application on his own behalf. The patient may be detained for up to 48 hours. After 48 hours, the patient is to be released unless he voluntarily consents to evaluation or treatment, or a proceeding for court-ordered evaluation or involuntary treatment is initiated.

A person may also be admitted as a voluntary patient if he makes application by express and informed consent, is shown to have evidence of mental illness, and is suitable for treatment. "Express and informed consent" is defined as "consent voluntarily given in writing after sufficient explanation and disclosure . . . to enable the person . . . to make a knowing and willful decision without any element of force, fraud, deceit, duress, or other form of constraint or coercion.[34] A voluntary patient may request discharge at any time and the facility administrator must either release him within three days or initiate the involuntary placement process.

In the court's discussion, it noted that "civil commitment for any purpose constitutes a significant deprivation of liberty that requires due process protection."[35] It is clear that a patient who is willing to sign forms but is incapable of making an informed decision is, by the same token, unlikely to benefit from the voluntary patient's statutory right to request discharge. As a result, the patient is in danger of being confined indefinitely without the benefit of the procedural safeguards of the involuntary placement process, which is specifically designed to protect persons incapable of looking after their own interests.

The physicians and staff at FSH were aware of the misuse of the voluntary admission process and to ensure that the proper procedure was followed. Thus, when they failed to provide constitutionally-required procedural safeguards to Mr. Burch, they deprived him of liberty, and cannot escape liability. As the court emphasized, "It is immaterial whether the due process violation Burch alleges is best described as arising from petitioners' (defendants') failure to comply with state procedures for admitting involuntary patients, or from the absence of a specific requirement that petitioners determine whether a patient is competent to consent to voluntary admission."[36]

The court concluded Mr. Burch was admitted to FSH in a way that did not ensure compliance with the statutory standard for voluntary admission. As the court concluded:

> The very risks created by the application of the informed-consent requirement to the special context of mental health care are borne out by the facts alleged in this case. It appears from the exhibits accompanying Burch's complaint that he was simply given admission forms to sign by clerical workers and, after he signed, was considered a voluntary patient. Burch alleges that petitioners knew or should have known that he was incapable of informed consent. This allegation is supported, at least as to petitioner Zimermon, by the psychiatrist's admission notes, described above, on Burch's mental state.[37]

---

34 *Id.* at 123.

35 *Id.* at 131.

36 *Id.* at 135–136.

37 *Id.* at 134.

SECTION 7-4: CLINICAL RESEARCH

In human research and experimentation, informed consent is a critical requirement to ensure that subjects are voluntary participants.

Two sets of Federal regulations affect clinical research using human subjects: one enacted by the Department of Health and Human Services (DHHS),[38], and the other by the Food and Drug Administration.[39] Under these regulations, review and approval by an institutional review board (IRB) is required for any experiment involving human subjects that is conducted by the DHHS or funded in whole or in part by it, or if non-FDA approved drugs are involved. These regulations focus in great depth on informed consent.

The Federal regulations specify in detail what information must be disclosed to prospective research subjects:

1. A statement that the study constitutes research, an explanation of its purposes and the expected duration of subject involvement, and a description of the procedures involved, with experimental procedures identified as such;
2. A description of risks and discomforts that are reasonably foreseeable;
3. A description of possible benefits to the subject and others;
4. Disclosure of appropriate alternative treatments, if any;
5. A statement describing the extent of confidentiality of medical records generated;
6. An explanation of whether compensation or treatment will be available if injuries occur;
7. A note as to who can be contacted with questions or reports of injury; and
8. A statement as to the voluntary nature of participation and the subject's right of withdrawal at any time.

There are also six *optional* elements of information that may be included if appropriate:

1. A statement that unforeseen risks may arise;
2. A description of circumstances in which the subject's participation may be terminated without the subject's consent;
3. A note as to any additional costs to the subject as a result of participation;

---

38 45 CFR Part 46.

39 21 CFR Part 50.

4. A description of the consequences of premature withdrawal;

5. A statement that subjects will be informed of any findings that may affect their willingness to continue; and

6. A notation of the number of subjects to be involved in the research.

SECTION 7-5: LIABILITIES

Various liabilities can result for failure to obtain consent or lack of informed consent. These may be criminal or civil actions, grounded in negligence or as an intentional tort.

If treatment is refused by a patient, there is no duty to provide treatment and no liability will arise for not treating the patient pursuant to that refusal. If treatment is provided *without* the patient's consent, there can be liability for battery. A battery is the unauthorized touching of a patient where there is no consent or consent has been revoked. There is greater potential for liability for refusing to honor the wishes of a patient than from complying with those wishes.

Lack of informed consent arises from an alleged failure to provide sufficient information to the patient so that an informed decision can be made. Consent to be touched has been given, thereby negating a battery, but it wasn't informed.

For a patient to prove lack of informed consent, the following elements are necessary:

1. Patient was injured by the procedure or treatment in question;

2. When the element not disclosed was a risk of treatment, the patient was injured by that specific risk; and

3. The patient must prove that, but for the failure to disclose, the patient would not have consented to the treatment or procedure.

Most courts have adopted an objective test to evaluate whether a reasonable person would have consented if that risk was known. A minority of courts use a subjective standard: would this particular patient have consented.

REFERENCES

Alt-White, A. C., *Obtaining 'Informed' Consent From the Elderly*, 17 Western Journal of Nursing Research 700 (December 1995).

Appelbaum, B. C., et al., *Competence To Consent to Voluntary Psychiatric Hospitalization: A Test of a Standard Proposed By APA*, 49 Psychiatric Services 1193 (September 1998).

Braddock, C. H., *Informed Decision Making in Outpatient Practice*, 282 JAMA 2313 (Dec 22/29, 1999).

Clayton, E. W., et al., *Informed Consent for Genetic Research on Stored Tissue Samples*, 274 JAMA 1786 (December 13, 1995).

Comeau, C. J., *The Nurse's Role in Informed Consent*, 1 Journal of Nursing Law 5 (Winter 1994).

DeRenzo, E. G., et al., *Assessment of Capacity To Give Consent To Research Participation: State-of-the-Art and Beyond*, 1 Journal of Health Care Law & Policy 66 (1998).

Karlawish, J. H. T., et al., *A Consensus-Based Approach To Providing Palliative Care To Patients Who Lack Decision-Making Capacity*, 130 Ann. Internal Med 835 (1999).

Kuczewski, M. G., *Reconceiving the Family: The Process of Consent in Medical Decisionmaking*, 26 Hastings Center Report 30 (March-April 1996).

Kurtz, S. F., *The Law of Informed Consent: From "Doctor is Right" to "Patient Has Rights,"* 50 Syracuse Law Review 1243 (2000).

Levine, E. G., et al., *Informed Consent: A Survey of Physician Outcomes and Practices,* 41 Gastrointestinal Endoscopy 448 (May 1995).

Liability/Professional Issues, 26 Mental & Physical Disability L. Rep. 888 (September/October 2002).

Rich, Ben A. *Prognostication In Clinical Medicine*, 23 J. Legal Med. 297 (September 2002).

Rosoff, A. J., *Informed Consent in the Electronic Age*, 25 American J. of Law & Medicine 367 (1999).

Schneider, C. E., *The Best-Laid Plans*, Hastings Center Rep. 24 (July-August 2000).

Stephenson, Joan, *Probing Informed Consent in Schizophrenia Research*, 281 JAMA 2273 (June 23/30, 1999).

Sugarman, J. et al., *Empirical Research on Informed Consent*, Hastings Center Report Supplement (January-February 1999).

Thomas, W. John, *Informed Consent, The Placebo Effect, and the Revenge of Thomas Percival*, 22 J. Legal Med 313 (2001).

CHAPTER 8

Treatment Decisions

by Jennifer Anne Marsh, Esq.[1]

SECTION 8-1: APPLICABLE LAWS AND ACCREDITATION STANDARDS

The Patient Self-Determination Act of 1990, which became effective December 1, 1991, is a powerful piece of legislation that mandates hospitals, skilled nursing facilities, home health agencies, hospice programs and prepaid organizations to advise patients of their legal rights and options to refuse or accept treatment. The primary purpose of this Act is to give adult patients an opportunity to learn about and use advance directives to set forth their treatment choices and to appoint surrogates if they lose decision-making capacity. The belief is that enhanced awareness and provision of information will promote discussions between patients and health care providers, and will likely result in patients completing advance directive documents. The primary provisions of the Act are as follows:

1. Patients must be offered written information regarding advance directives and all adult patients must be given summaries of pertinent institutional policies regarding their rights under state and federal law to accept or refuse treatment and to make advance directives.

---

1 Jennifer Anne Marsh, Esq. received her Bachelor's of Journalism, *cum laude*, from the University of Missouri—Columbia in 2000. Ms. Marsh received her Juris Doctorate, *cum laude,* and Health Law Certificate from Saint Louis University in 2003. While in law school, Ms. Marsh was the Editor-in-Chief of the *Journal of Health Law*, and received an Academic Excellence Award in Bioethics. Ms. Marsh now practices as an Associate in the Health Care Business Law Group of Shughart Thomson & Kilroy, P.C. in Kansas City, Missouri.

2. There must be documentation in the patient's record to indicate whether the patient has any advance directives.

3. Institutions may not discriminate against or condition care provided to a patient on the basis of whether the patient has executed any advance directives.

4. Institutions have an affirmative obligation to comply with requirements of state and federal law regarding advance directives.

5. Institutions must provide individually or with others education to staff and to the community regarding issues associated with advance directives.

In 1995, a study was conducted evaluating the extent to which patients discussed and prepared advance directives after being exposed to a program that responded to the requirements of the Patient Self-Determination Act. The study concluded there was limited effectiveness of the hospital's advance directive program. There was only modest compliance with the implementation of the program. Thirty percent of the patients were never asked by a nurse whether they had an advance directive, and forty-three percent of the patients never received the brochure. Only fifty-seven percent of those patients who were asked about advance directives remembered the inquiry, demonstrating that many of the nurse-patient interactions had a limited effect on enhancing patient awareness of advance directives.

Several suggestions have been made to enhance the effectiveness of the program. Nurses must receive more education on advance directives as well as be given more time to effectively discuss this subject matter with their patients. Follow-up discussions on advance directives should occur at a later time in the patient's hospitalization. The lack of time during the admission process and information overload may preclude retention of information and prevent adequate discussions. Advance directive programs also need to be sensitive to the cultural diversity of their patient population, as different ethnic and racial groups have diverse perceptions of the concept of advance planning. Active rather than passive means of disseminating information need to be employed to enhance patient knowledge. Brochures need to be written at the lowest level of comprehension of a significant portion of the patient population.[2]

Advance directive documents must be placed in patients' medical records and their provisions implemented. Some provisions may have to be effected by having orders from a physician if required by facility policy, such as do-not-resuscitate directives. Yet a nurse is subject to liability for providing treatment

---

2 Silverman, H. J., *et al. Implementation of the Patient Self-Determination Act in a Hospital Setting: An Initial Evaluation*, 155 Archives of Internal Medicine 502 (March 13, 1995).

without consent which may arise if the nurse is aware of the patient's directives but refuses to follow them without an order. This places the nurse in a serious legal and ethical dilemma.

More recent laws also have attempted to promote the use of advance directives. In 1999, Federal regulations established a patients' rights Condition of Participation in Medicare that applies to hospitals. The regulations require that each patient be informed of his health status, be involved in care planning and treatment, and be able to request or refuse treatment. The regulations also state that each patient has a right to draft an advance directive, and that patients have the right to have hospital staff and practitioners comply with the advance directives.[3] A hospital's Medicare funding could be jeopardized for failure to comply with these regulations.

Intractable pain is another topic that has been the focus of many lawmakers, with many states adopting intractable pain relief acts. These state laws generally promote access to drug therapy for patients who suffer from chronic or intractable pain. Many of these laws shield practitioners who prescribe pain medication from criminal investigation and state licensing board scrutiny. The laws may require a practitioner to consult with a pain specialist prior to prescribing the medication, to meticulously document the administration of the medication, and to document the intractable pain in the medical record.

In addition to the attention they have received from lawmakers, treatment issues also have been the focus of recent revisions to accreditation standards. Most health care institutions will seek accreditation from a private health care organization. Although accreditation technically is voluntary, as a practical matter accreditation may be necessary for a provider to meet Medicare certification requirements or state licensure standards. The leading private accreditation institution, the Joint Commission on Accreditation of Healthcare Organizations (JCAHO), has developed a number of accreditation standards that could impact treatment decisions.

First, JCAHO Standard R1.2.30 in the *Comprehensive Accreditation Manual for Hospitals* requires that patients be involved in decisions about care, treatment, and services provided. The standard recognizes that conflicts and dilemmas will arise for the patient, family members and other decision makers regarding the admission, care, treatment, services or discharge of the patient, and the standard requires that the hospital work with the patients and their families to resolve these dilemmas. This standard is often met by institutional ethics committees that help to resolve conflicts regarding the appropriate course of treatment.

---

3   42 C.F.R. § 482.13(b)(2).

Second, JCAHO Standard RI.2.80 provides that the hospital must address the wishes of the patient regarding end-of-life decisions. Under this standard, the hospital must have in place policies regarding advance directives, the withdrawal or life-sustaining treatment, and withholding resuscitation services. Adults must be given written information about these policies, and whether or not the patient has signed an advance directive must be documented in the medical record. The standard mandates that hospital staff be aware of the advance directive, if one exists, and that care providers honor advance directives within the limits of the law and the hospital's capabilities.

Finally, the JCAHO standards recognize that patients have the right to pain management. Standard RI.2.160 requires that "the hospital plans, supports, and coordinates activities and resources to ensure that pain is recognized and addressed appropriately and in accordance with the care, treatment and services provided . . . ."

SECTION 8-2: TREATMENT DECISIONS REGARDING MINORS AND NEWBORNS

Many judicial decisions address the issue of whether and under what circumstance parental autonomy in making treatment decisions for their children may be overridden by courts. Courts have embraced the doctrine of *parens patriae*, or the right of the state to intervene when the health and safety of a child is in jeopardy, to justify overriding parents' decisions regarding the medical treatment of their children. Federal and state courts have unhesitatingly authorized medical treatment over a parent's objection in situations where treatment is relatively innocuous in comparison to the dangers of withholding medical care. For example, numerous cases have overridden the religious objections of parents to life-saving, safe, and necessary blood transfusions for their minor children. These cases reason that, because the transfusion is ordered by the court and is not the willful decision of the parents, the parents should not consider themselves in violation of their religious beliefs.

Some cases, however, have examined the best interests of the child, and upheld parents' decisions to refuse treatment for their children. *Newmark v. Williams*[4], involved a three year old child with pediatric lymphoma. The child's parents, who were devout Christian Scientists, rejected all forms of treatment for their child and refused to authorize chemotherapy. In deciding not to declare the child "neglected" under a state statute, the court closely examined the best interests of the child, and found that the state's authority to intervene did not out-

---

4 588 A.2d 1108 (Del. Supr. 1991).

weigh the parental prerogative to refuse treatment for the child. In upholding the parents' decision to refuse treatment, the court noted that:

The egregious facts of this case indicate that [the child's] proposed medical treatment was highly invasive, painful, involved terrible temporary and potentially permanent side effects, posed an unacceptably low chance of success, and a high risk that the treatment itself would cause his death.[5]

Modern cases indicate that the best approach for a practitioner who wants to override a parent's decision regarding a child's medical condition is to instigate child protective proceedings, as was done in the *Newmark* case. Most states' child abuse and neglect statutes provide that parents' failure to provide adequate health care for their child constitutes neglect. Under these statutes, the state can obtain legal custody of the children, and ensure that the necessary treatment is provided.

. On October 9, 1984, Congress enacted the Child Abuse Amendments of 1984 to the Child Abuse Prevention and Treatment Act.[6] These amendments redefined "child abuse" to include medical neglect. Additionally, "medically indicated treatment" may not be withheld from disabled infants with life-threatening conditions. Treatment must be provided that in the physician's reasonable medical judgment would be most likely to correct life-threatening conditions. The amendments do provide that treatment may be withheld if the infant is chronically and irreversibly comatose, if the treatment would be futile or would merely prolong dying, or if treatment would cause substantial pain and suffering to the infant. The regulations condition states' receipt of federal child abuse prevention funding on the existence of procedures to deal with reports of infant neglect.

SECTION 8-3: ADVANCE DIRECTIVES

Advance directives are mechanisms to allow individuals, while they are still competent, to make known their decisions regarding health care treatment that may be required in the future. They only become effective when the individual lacks capacity at the time that a specific decision needs to be made. Advance directives may be written or oral. While there are no legal barriers to upholding oral advance directives, there may be potential problems in verifying their applicability to a given situation. Thus, it is usually in the patient's best interest to put advance directives in writing. Additionally, any communications from a patient about future treatment decisions should be clearly documented in the patient's medical record, using the patient's own words as much as remembered.

---

5 *Id.* at 1118.

6 42 U.S.C. § 5101 *et seq.*

The majority of states have enacted legislation defining specific advance directives and the required criteria for their execution. Even if a state does not have such legislation, however, advance directives, both in writing and verbal, still have at least the force of moral directives to health care providers and courts.

Advance directives provide two important functions. First, they clearly indicate the patient's choices about treatment decisions, thereby ensuring respect for the patient's autonomy. Second, advance directives allow health care providers to follow the patient's personal directives without seeking court intervention.

Advance directives do not always resolve what course of action is appropriate because patients and families often waiver when confronted with imminent death. It is also frequently difficult to predict whether an emergency intervention will improve the patient's quality of life or limit the patient to a long, painful process of high-tech dying. Yet it is clear that health care providers and facilities often do not consider advance directives and patient wishes when making treatment decisions.

This failure to honor advance directives may create a significant risk of legal liability for health care providers. The first case in which a provider had to pay significant damages for failure to honor an advance directive involved a patient who suffered from violent seizures. The patient, Brenda Young, needed total care, and had to be fed, bathed, diapered and tied to her bed at night to avoid pushing herself over her padded bed rails. Sometimes Ms. Young managed a few intelligible words, such as "water" or "bury me."

Warned that the seizures from which she had long suffered were likely to worsen, Ms. Young gave her mother power of attorney to stop treatment if she became incapacitated. Despite this, after her next seizure, Ms. Young was put on a ventilator, tube fed, and maintained through a two-month coma, over her mother's insistence that she did not want life support. This was precisely the kind of existence that Ms. Young had sought to avoid by signing an advance directive one month before the seizure that left her so disabled. In a lawsuit against the hospital, Ms. Young and her mother won a $16.5 million verdict.[7]

Although this case is apparently the first in which a jury has awarded substantial damages, it is clear there is an increasing number of lawsuits seeking to hold health care providers and facilities liable for failing to honor advance directives. In the 1999 case of *Klavan v. Crozer-Chester Medical Center*[8], a court considered a constitutional law challenge to a care provider's disregard of an advance directive. The patient in this case had adopted an advance directive that

---

7 Lewin, T., *Ignoring 'Right to Die' Directives, Medical Community is Being Sued*, The New York Times 1 (June 2, 1996).

8 60 F.Supp. 2d. 436 (E.D. Pa. 1999).

instructed attending physicians "to withhold or withdraw treatment that merely prolongs my dying" in the event of an incurable or irreversible condition, such as a coma, persistent vegetative state, and brain damage or brain disease. Four years after adopting the advance directive, the patient, himself a physician, attempted suicide, and left a note near where he was found indicating that he did not want to be resuscitated. Despite this, the defendants, a hospital and individual physicians, undertook extreme medical measures and successfully resuscitated the patient. Several weeks later, the patient suffered a massive stroke and was declared totally incapacitated.

Thereafter, the patient, through his guardian *ad litem*, brought suit on several theories. First, the patient's attorneys argued that failure to honor the advance directive was a breach of contract. Second, they argued that failure to obtain the patient's consent was a medical battery. Finally, the patient's suit cited the Fourteenth Amendment's Due Process Clause, and argued that the defendants' actions violated the patient's constitutionally protected liberty interest in refusing unwanted medical treatment.

A United States District Court sitting in Pennsylvania, however, dismissed this lawsuit on the grounds that there was no state action, or governmental transgression, as is required to sue under the Fourteenth Amendment's Due Process Clause.[9] The court ruled that the defendants were private actors, and that their disregard of the advance directive could not be considered state action merely because the defendants received Medicaid funds and a state license.

The legal theories in cases involving practitioners who fail to honor advance directives vary, with some based on negligence, some alleging that treatment against the patient's will is a battery, some asserting constitutional violations, and others arguing intentional infliction of emotional, physical and financial distress. Health care providers and facilities must be acutely aware of their potential risk when failing to honor a patient's advance directive.

SECTION 8-4: BRAIN DEATH

Historically, the loss of heart and lung functions was easily observable and a sufficient basis for diagnosing death. With the advent of effective artificial cardiopulmonary support for severely brain-injured persons, confusion has been created regarding the determination of death. Despite the loss of all brain functions, circulation and respiration can be maintained with a mechanical respirator and other medical interventions.

To reliably be able to recognize that death has occurred, accurate criteria must be defined. These criteria should:

---

9 *Id.* at 445.

1. eliminate errors in classifying a living individual as dead;
2. allow as few errors as possible in classifying a dead body as alive;
3. allow a determination to be made without unreasonable delay;
4. be adaptable to a variety of clinical situations; and
5. be explicit and accessible to verification.[10]

Recognizing the need for a uniform definition of death, the American Bar Association, American Medical Association, the National Conference of Commissioners on Uniform State Laws, and the President's Commission for the Study of Ethical Problems in Medicine and Biomedical and Behavioral Research proposed the following model statute for determination of death:

An individual who has sustained either (1) irreversible cessation of circulatory and respiratory functions, or (2) irreversible cessation of all functions of the entire brain, including the brain stem, is dead. A determination of death must be made in accordance with accepted medical standards.

To determine cardiopulmonary death requires clinical examination to disclose the absence of responsiveness, heart beat, and respiratory effort. These generally are determinations within the knowledge of nurses; therefore, the determination of cardiopulmonary death may be made by a nurse. In some instances, medical circumstances may require the use of confirmatory tests such as an EKG.

To determine neurological death, that there is cerebral unreceptivity and unresponsivity, usually requires confirmatory studies such as an EEG or blood flow study. The tests used to determine cessation of brain functions are changing with the advent of new research and technologies. Thus, nurses should rely on "accepted medical standards," which will reflect current practice.

Reliable testing of brain stem reflexes requires an experienced physician using adequate stimuli. Most difficulties with the determination of death based on neurological criteria result from inadequate attention to the cause of the coma and the possibility of recovery of any brain function. The duration of the observation period for making these determinations is within the clinical judgment of the physician.

The vast majority of States have accepted death as defined by either the cardiopulmonary test or neurological test. This allows uniformity among the States which is extremely beneficial, especially in the area of organ transplantation and donation.

---

10 *Guidelines for the Determination of Death*, 246 JAMA 2184 (Nov. 13, 1981).

SECTION 8-5: MEDICAL FUTILITY

Treatment is regarded as medically futile when it has no reasonable chance of achieving a therapeutic benefit for the patient. Treatment that is medically futile does not have to be offered or provided to the patient. Health care providers are charged with the determination of medical futility. Medical futility issues often arise in cases where patients demand treatment that is not indicated or would be therapeutically useless.

Few cases involving questions of medical futility have been litigated; however, a majority of the cases that have been decided have found in favor of the patient, and allowed a medically futile treatment to continue. For example, in *In re Conservatorship of Wanglie*[11], the court considered the case of an eighty-five year old patient, who was first admitted to the hospital after falling in her home and fracturing her hip. For several months after her admission, the patient suffered many serious medical events, such as cardiopulmonary arrest, which left her in a persistent vegetative state. The patient was receiving aggressive treatment at the request of her husband, who demanded the treatment be continued in contravention of the opinion of the attending physicians and the hospital's medical ethicist. The hospital sought to appoint a conservator to determine the patient's best interest. The trial court, however, appointed the patient's husband, who had demanded the futile treatment continue, as conservator, reasoning he was best able to act on behalf of the patient.

Another representative case of medical futility is *In re Baby K.*[12] In this case, an anencephalic infant presented to the emergency department in respiratory distress. The infant's physicians argued that placing the infant on a ventilator was medically and ethically inappropriate, and that the prevailing standard of care for infants with anencephaly is to provide only warmth, nutrition, and hydration. The court, however, ruled that respiratory distress is an emergency under the Emergency Medical Treatment and Active Labor Act (EMTALA), and held that the hospital was obligated to provide respiratory support to the infant.[13]

The American Medical Association (AMA) has addressed medical futility in its Code of Ethics, which allows physicians to decline to provide futile treatments. The AMA standard on futility, states that:

> Physicians are not ethically obligated to deliver care that, in their best professional judgment, will not have a reasonable chance of benefitting their patients. Patients should not be given treatments simply

---

11 No. PX-91-283 (D. Minn. P. Div. July 1, 1991).

12 16 F.3d 590 (4th Cir. 1994).

13 *Id.* at 594–595.

because they demand them. Denial of treatment should be justified by reliance on openly stated ethical principles and acceptable standards of care. . . .[14]

The AMA also requires all health care institutions to adopt a policy on medical futility, and has drafted the following seven steps, which should be assessed when declaring a treatment to be futile:

1. Earnest attempts should be made in advance to deliberate over and negotiate prior understandings between patient, proxy and physician on what constitutes futile care for the patient, and what falls within acceptable limits for the physician, family, and possibly also the institution.
2. Joint decision-making should occur between patient or proxy and physician to the maximum extent possible.
3. Attempts should be made to negotiate disagreements if they arise, and to reach resolution within all parties' acceptable limits, with the assistance of consultants as appropriate.
4. Involvement of an institutional committee such as the ethics committee should be requested if disagreements are irresolvable.
5. If the institutional review supports the patient's position and the physician remains unpersuaded, transfer of care to another physician within the institution may be arranged.
6. If the process supports the physician's position and the patient/proxy remains unpersuaded, transfer to another institution may be sought and, if done, should be supported by the transferring and receiving institution.
7. If transfer is not possible, the intervention need not be offered.[15]

Most hospitals have developed futility policies in compliance with the AMA Opinions. Some critics, however, have argued that futility policies are merely a way to cut medical costs by rationing care.

Courts have also responded to the argument that declining futile treatment undermines the medical profession. For example, in *Superintendent of Belchertown State School v. Saikewicz*[16], the court noted that:

> [p]revailing medical ethical practice does not, without exception, demand that all efforts toward life prolongation be made in all circumstances. . . . Recognition of the right to refuse necessary treatment in

---

14 AMA Council on Ethical and Judicial Affairs, *Opinion E-2.035* (1994).

15 AMA Council on Ethical and Judicial Affairs, *Opinion E-2.037.*

16 370 N.E.2d 417 (Mass. 1977).

appropriate circumstances is consistent with existing medical mores; such a doctrine does not threaten either the integrity of the medical profession, the proper role of hospitals in caring for such patients or the State's interest in protecting the same.[17]

SECTION 8-6: DO-NOT-RESUSCITATE/NO-CODE-BLUE ORDERS

Do-not-resuscitate/no-code-blue orders have long been a source of conflict and frustration for nurses. Frequently physicians have not honored a patient's right not to be resuscitated and have failed to write an appropriate order or have verbally advised the nurses to perform a "slow code." A decision regarding resuscitation is a moral decision belonging to the patient, not a medical, nursing or legal decision, although those perspectives are important considerations for the patient. If the patient lacks the capacity to make the decision, it then should be made by the court appointed guardian, surrogate, or family in conjunction with the attending and any appropriate consulting physicians, nurses, and other staff.

While it is clear that patients are entitled to make informed decisions regarding cardiopulmonary resuscitation, which includes a discussion of the prognosis and the risks and benefits of CPR, the data suggest that physicians often don't discuss CPR with patients at all.[18] Yet the information about the effects and outcomes of CPR is an important determinant in the decisions patients make regarding CPR. Patients base their decisions for life support on perceived outcomes, and those patients who are most informed about CPR outcomes were more likely to reject CPR. Interestingly, patients consistently overestimated their CPR survival chances. An explanation for this is that most patients reported learning about CPR from television, which often depicts CPR as successful.

Do-not-resuscitate/no-code-blue orders are legal and binding. They must be justified, however, either as a patient request or when medically indicated. The decision whether to write a do-not-resuscitate/no-code-blue order must be based upon well-established criteria.

The issue in *Payne v. Marion General Hospital*[19], was whether the patient was competent at the time a no-code order was issued. Mr. Payne was a sixty-five year old alcoholic who had allowed his condition to deteriorate to the point he required hospitalization. He was admitted to the hospital suffering from mal-

---

17 *Id.* at 426–427.

18 Schonwetter, R.S., et al., *Resuscitation Decision Making in the Elderly: The Value of Outcome Data*, 8 Journal of General Internal Medicine 295 (June 1993).

19 549 N.E.2d 1043 (Ind. App. 2nd Dist. 1990).

nutrition, uremia, hypertensive cardiovascular disease, chronic obstructive lung disease, non-union of a previously fractured left humerus, and congenital levoscoliosis of the lumbar spine. Throughout his hospitalization, his condition worsened as his temperature rose and his respirations became more frequent and labored. He became congested and mucous was aspirated from his lungs.

Mr. Payne's sister informed the nurse she did not want Mr. Payne resuscitated if he began to die. The nurse contacted Mr. Payne's treating physician and informed him of Mr. Payne's condition and of his sister's request. After consulting with the nurse and talking to Mr. Payne's sister, the treating physician authorized the entry of a no-code order on Mr. Payne's chart. Mr. Payne's condition continued to worsen and he subsequently had a cardiac arrest and died because no cardiopulmonary resuscitation was attempted.

The testimony of all the nurses who attended to Mr. Payne was that he was conscious, alert, and able to communicate when the no-code order was entered and that he remained competent until shortly before his death. As the court noted: "The patient's right of self-determination is the *sine qua non* of the physician's duty to obtain informed consent."[20] Thus, Mr. Payne's treating physician had a duty to obtain his consent prior to entering the no-code order.

Documentation in the medical record supporting a do-not-resuscitate/no-code-blue order must include at least the following:

1. The process leading to the patient's current condition;
2. An estimation of the patient's prognosis and reversibility of the condition;
3. A summary of the discussions, identifying with whom; and
4. Who authorized the do not resuscitate/no code blue order.

When a decision is made to not resuscitate, most health care facilities require that to be given as an order by a physician. Telephone or verbal orders should be permissible unless prohibited by state law.

In *Anderson v. St. Francis-St. George Hospital*[21], the administrator of the estate of a deceased patient brought suit against the hospital, alleging battery, negligence, and wrongful living. On May 25, 1988, Edward Winter was admitted to the hospital suffering chest pain. Mr. Winter had a discussion with his family and his physician, Dr. Russo, about the type of treatment that he was to receive while at the hospital. As a result of that discussion, Dr. Russo entered a no-code-blue order in his hospital record.

---

20 *Id.* at 1046.

21 614 N.E.2d 841 (Ohio App. 1st Dist. 1992).

On May 28, Mr. Winter suffered a ventricular fibrillation. Despite Dr. Russo's order, a nurse resuscitated Mr. Winter by defibrillation. The nurse's resuscitation prevented Mr. Winter's natural death and was a battery to Mr. Winter. The nurse was alleged to be negligent by resuscitating Mr. Winter contrary to Dr. Russo's order. By keeping Mr. Winter alive, the hospital caused him "great pain, suffering, emotional distress and disability" as well as medical and other financial expenses.

When a health care provider treats a patient without consent, that constitutes a battery. If a patient has expressly refused treatment, even in an emergency, any medical treatment is a battery.[22] The evidence was clear that Mr. Winter had expressly refused treatment in a code blue situation. There was no disagreement that defibrillation was within the ambit of Dr. Russo's no-code-blue order. The court thus concluded that the hospital committed a battery to Mr. Winter in resuscitating him.

The issue then became what harm was proximately caused by the hospital's wrongful act. Mr. Winter had damages after the defibrillation that included a paralyzing stroke, pain, suffering, emotional distress and disability, and medical expenses. It was thus a question for the jury as to whether these damages were proximately caused by the hospital's wrongful act.

Do-not-resuscitate/no-code-blue orders should be reconsidered periodically according to changes in the patient's clinical status. Any required time period for review and/or renewal of the order should be specified in the policy.

An issue that has been significantly ignored is whether DNR orders should be honored during the perioperative period. Should DNR orders be treated like most medical orders, i.e., rescinded prior to surgery and rewritten in the postoperative period? Or should DNR orders remain effective throughout surgery and recovery? These questions invoke challenging issues that must be carefully considered. If the policy is to override DNR orders during surgery, patients are then put in the difficult position of having to weigh the benefits of surgery against the risks of unwanted resuscitation. If DNR orders are to be honored during the perioperative period, however, surgeons and anesthesiologists are restrained from correcting complications for which they may be legally responsible.

The Association of Operating Nurses has issued a position statement regarding perioperative care of patients with DNR orders. Its position is as follows:

> A DNR order should not mean that all treatment is stopped and the need for medical and nursing care is eliminated, but rather that the patient has made certain choices about end-of-life decisions. A patient's rights do not stop at the entrance to the operating room.

---

22 *Id.* at 844.

Automatically suspending a DNR order during surgery undermines a patient's right to self-determination. Development of a policy related to DNR orders in the operating room is supported by the Patient Self-Determination Act, the Joint Commission on Accreditation of Healthcare Organizations (JCAHO), the "ANA Code for Nurses with Interpretive Statements—Explications for Perioperative Nursing," and *A Patient's Bill of Rights*.[23]

If the policy of a health care facility is to suspend all DNR orders during the perioperative period, patients at least must be made aware of this policy. Legal precedent suggests that patients must be notified of such a policy at the time of admission to the facility.

Another issue related to DNR orders that is rarely discussed is limited resuscitative efforts or partial codes. Although there is no standard definition of "partial code," it is generally considered a situation in which a patient receives some, but not all, of the elements of cardiopulmonary resuscitation. A "slow code" is typically a verbal order either to respond slowly to an arrest or to respond to the code as usual but to call the physician when the arrest occurs to obtain further direction. These codes have been described as shades of code blue: "light blue," "sky blue," "navy blue, " and "dark blue," depending on how much CPR is involved. Dr. Goldenring asserted that: "The partial code represents a tempting act of rationalization that is neither medically or ethically sound . . . I doubt that 'partial codes' can be justified, but I see them frequently. . . ."[24]

In 1983, the President's Commission for the Study of Ethical Problems in Medicine and Biomedical and Behavioral Research viewed partial codes negatively. "Success at resuscitation is rare enough when all efforts are expended, so such limited efforts are usually doomed from the start." The President's Commission concluded that "Partial codes were conducted from a desire to deceive the patient or family, usually due to the physician's discomfort in discussing the patient's imminent death. A partial code was instituted to make it look as if everything possible was being done, even though the physician knew or believed that resuscitation was not warranted given the circumstances."[25]

A partial code that intends to deceive a patient or the family cannot be justified. From a medical and legal perspective, a patient generally should have either full resuscitation or no resuscitation.

---

23 Association of Operating Room Nurses, Inc. *Position Statement: Perioperative Care of Patients with Do Not Resuscitate Orders* (1995).

24 Goldenring, J., *Correspondence,* 300 New England Journal of Medicine 1057 (1979).

25 The President's Commission for the Study of Ethical Problems in Medicine and Biomedical and Behavioral Research, *Deciding to Forego Life-Sustaining Treatment* (1983).

SECTION 8-7: WITHHOLDING / WITHDRAWING TREATMENT

The corollary to an individual's right to consent to health care treatment is that the individual has the right to refuse to consent or to withdraw consent at any time. This is based upon the common law right of freedom from nonconsensual invasion of one's body, along with the constitutional right of privacy.

This right to refuse health care treatment extends to life-saving and life-prolonging care, regardless of the patient's underlying condition. A patient may refuse treatment even for a non-terminal condition. When a patient who has the capacity to make a health care decision requests the withholding or withdrawal of any health care treatment, there is no duty to contact or seek input of family members or next of kin. The *patient* retains the sole right to make that decision.

In our society, due to great advances in medical knowledge and technology over the last few decades, death does not come suddenly or completely unexpectedly to most people. While medical advances have made it possible to forestall and cure certain illnesses, the result is to prolong the slow deterioration and death of some patients and to hold them on the threshold of death for an indeterminate period of time. As a result, questions of fate have become matters of choice raising profound moral, social, technological, philosophical, and legal issues involving the interplay of many disciplines. When a patient decides to withhold or withdraw treatment, it must first be determined that the patient has the capacity at that time to make that health care decision. This evaluation is to be made by the appropriate health care providers and should be documented in the medical record. Next it should be ascertained that information about the patient's condition, prognosis, the alternative treatments available, and the risks involved in the withholding or withdrawal of treatment has been adequately explained to the patient. Finally it must be verified that the patient made that treatment choice voluntarily and without coercion. Provided these criteria are met, courts have repeatedly held that an adult has the right to refuse any health care treatment.

Tort liability may arise for nonconsensual touching even if it is deemed to be in the patient's best interest. There is a growing body of commentary and legal decisions favoring a patient's right to die over any legal, medical, or political objections. Lawsuits have been initiated and won against health care providers and institutions for damages arising from providing treatment to a patient without consent.

In a case based on a tort claim for nonconsensual touching, a court held that a physician was subject to liability for wrongfully placing and maintaining a patient on a respirator. In *Estate of Leach v. Shapiro*[26], the patient's family filed

---

26 469 N.E.2d 1047 (Ohio App. 1984).

a lawsuit seeking damages for placing Mrs. Leach on a life support system without her consent or the consent of her family. The patient suffered a respiratory and cardiac arrest. She had expressly advised defendants that she did not wish to be kept alive by machines. The family sought damages for invasion of privacy, pain and suffering, mental anguish, special damages for the cost of unnecessary and unwanted medical care, and punitive damages. The court held that a physician who treats a patient without consent commits a battery, although the procedure is harmless or even beneficial. In this case, a cause of action existed for wrongfully placing and maintaining the patient on a life support system contrary to the expressed wishes of the patient and family.

The rights of privacy and self-determination, i.e. the rights to make treatment choices, are not lost merely because a patient loses the capacity to exercise those decisions. This has been repeatedly recognized by courts throughout the country. It was first discussed by the New Jersey Supreme Court in *Matter of Quinlan*[27], As the court reasoned:

> If a putative decision by Karen to permit this non-cognitive, vegetative existence to terminate by natural forces is regarded as a valuable incident of her right of privacy, as we believe it to be, then it should not be discarded solely on the basis that her condition prevents her conscious exercise of the choice.[28]

Courts have cited the Equal Protection Clause of the Fourteenth Amendment as authority for the proposition that incompetent patients still have a right to refuse or withdraw treatment. Under this approach, courts have noted that the decision whether or not to refuse care may be made by a proxy acting on behalf of an incompetent patient.

If the patient lacks capacity to consent to health care treatment decisions, only a court appointed guardian or other legally authorized person may give consent. While some states have statutes authorizing consent from family members or next of kin, the majority of states have traditionally relied upon this custom without any legal authority. More frequently, it is a legal issue because treatment decisions made by non-legally authorized persons can be challenged by others, exposing health care providers and facilities to potential legal liability for acting without authorized consent.

The law historically has permitted people to designate others to act on their behalf using the device known as the power of attorney. When an individual authorizes a power of attorney, he can name another person who is legally authorized to sign documents, conduct transactions, or take other actions on that

---

27 355 A.2d 647 (N.J. 1976).

28 *Id.* at 664.

person's behalf. Traditionally, those actions were limited to business and financial transactions. Only in a few states has it been expressly stated that the power of delegation is applicable to decisions affecting health care treatment. Thus, many commentators and health care attorneys take the position that there is no authority through the power of attorney to make health care treatment decisions.

Many states have now adopted laws that allow an individual to designate a surrogate to act as a substitute decision-maker when the individual lacks the capacity to make health care treatment decisions. While a few states have adopted laws limiting the scope of a surrogate's authority, the majority of courts have adopted an approach that gives the surrogate the same authority that the patient would have if competent. Additionally, the surrogate is allowed to exercise those rights without judicial involvement even if it involves refusing treatment or life-prolonging care.

While accepting the rights of an incompetent patient to autonomy and self-determination, two standards have developed for decision-making by a surrogate to exercise those rights. They are "substituted judgment" and "best interest."

The substituted judgment standard seeks to preserve the autonomy of the patient and endeavors to reach the same decision that the patient would make at that time if the patient had the capacity to do so. This requires considering those factors and circumstances the patient would use in making that health care treatment decision. A substituted judgment advances the values of the individual's autonomy and self-determination, which are the underlying bases for informed consent. It preserves to the extent possible the dignity and respect for the individual.

If a patient has clearly expressed personal intentions about medical treatment, they will be respected. Where the intentions are not definitive, the "substituted judgment" approach best accomplishes the goal of making the same decision that the patient would make if capable at that time. This requires that the surrogate decision-maker consider the patient's personal value system, prior statements about and reactions to medical issues, and all the facets of the patient's personality with which the surrogate is familiar. Particular reference should be made to relevant philosophical, theological, and ethical values in order to extrapolate what course of medical treatment the patient would choose. *Matter of Jobes.*[29]

Courts repeatedly have adopted and applied the substituted judgment standard whenever possible rather than alternative standards for proxy decision-making. Only this approach permits the genuine exercise of the incompetent's right to self-determination.

---

29 529 A.2d 434, 444 (N.J. 1987).

The "best interest" standard is based on the ethical principle of beneficence and seeks to make decisions that benefit the patient. It requires an objective assessment of what will promote the patient's welfare, without reference to the patient's previously-stated or supposed preference. To arrive at a best interest decision requires considering the following objective criteria:

1. Relief from suffering;
2. Preservation or restoration of functioning;
3. Quality and extent of sustained life;
4. Satisfaction of present desires;
5. Opportunities for future satisfactions; and
6. The possibility of developing or regaining capacity for self-determination.

Even using the best interest standard, a choice may be made to refuse further life-prolonging care because that is determined to be in the patient's best interest. This standard does not require endless or useless treatment. However, when a patient has any degree of awareness, i.e., is not in a persistent vegetative state, courts usually conclude that the potential for even limited participation and awareness is preferable to death.

In cases involving treatment decisions regarding terminally ill patients or patients in a persistent vegetative state, courts have never imposed life-prolonging treatment on a patient in opposition to the patient's expressed wishes or a substituted judgment. Courts have upheld a patient's right to refuse artificial respiration, dialysis, IV medications, amputations, and artificial nutrition. Courts have, however, placed restrictions upon the process by which decisions may be made.

The only exception to adherence to a patient's right of self-determination in health care treatment decisions is when the state's interest is determined superior to the patient's wishes. The state's interests are defined as:

1. Preserving life;
2. Preventing suicide;
3. Protecting innocent third parties; and
4. Maintaining the ethical standards of the health care profession.

Because a patient's right to refuse treatment is not absolute, it must be balanced against these four countervailing interests. In most instances, courts will uphold a patient's right to refuse treatment unless some third party is involved, which consistently has been viewed as a significant interest. For example, courts have limited the right to refuse treatment for contagious diseases, pregnant women, and parents of small children.

While courts traditionally have respected the right of Jehovah's Witnesses to refuse blood transfusions, they have rejected that right when a parent wants to deny a transfusion to a minor child. Other courts have overridden that right when it could cause harm to a third party.

There is no meaningful distinction between withdrawing and withholding life-prolonging care or any treatment. Stopping treatment requires no greater justification than not starting treatment. While some argue that discontinuing life-sustaining treatment is an "active" taking of life as opposed to the more "passive" act of omitting treatment in the first instance, such argument is without legal support. As the New Jersey Supreme Court stated in *Matter of Conroy:*

> This distinction is more psychologically compelling than logically sound. As mentioned above, the line between active and passive conduct in the context of medical decisions is far too nebulous to constitute a principled basis for decision-making . . . Moreover, from a policy standpoint, it might well be unwise to forbid persons from discontinuing a treatment under circumstances in which the treatment could permissibly be withheld. Such a rule could discourage families and doctors from even attempting certain types of care and could thereby force them into hasty and premature decisions to allow a patient to die.[30]

In deciding whether it is appropriate to terminate life support for a patient, determine that the patient is in a persistent vegetative state with no likelihood of restoration to cognitive or sapient life. This is defined as the capacity to maintain the vegetative parts of neurological function without any cognitive function. A patient has no awareness of anything or anyone and exists at a primitive reflex level. Although there may be some brain stem function and other reactions one normally associates with being alive, such as moving, reacting to light, sound and noxious stimuli, and blinking of the eyes, the quality of the feeling impulses is unknown. No form of treatment which can cure or improve this condition is known or available. The prognosis is extremely poor and the extent of any recovery unknown if it should, in fact, occur.

Diagnosing a patient as being in a persistent vegetative state is not a simple procedure. In *Matter of Quinlan*[31], the court felt it was important to free physicians from possible contamination by self-interest or self-protection concerns which would inhibit their independent medical judgments for the well-being of their dying patients. The court suggested that it would be more appro-

---

30 *Matter of Conroy*, 486 A.2d 1209, 1234 (N.J. 1985).

31 355 A.2d 647 (N.J. 1976).

priate to provide a regular forum for more input and dialogue in individual situations and to allow the responsibility of these judgments to be shared.

The court identified an ethics committee composed of physicians, social workers, attorneys, and theologians as an appropriate panel to review the individual circumstances of ethical dilemmas and to provide assistance and safeguards for patients and their medical caretakers. In effect, the court was focusing on a prognosis committee to provide a mechanism to confirm the diagnosis and prognosis of an individual patient and minimize the necessity of seeking judicial intervention. As the court concluded: "Decision-making within health care if it is considered as an expression of a primary obligation of the physician . . . should be controlled primarily within the patient-doctor-family relationship. . . ."[32]

SECTION 8-8: ARTIFICIAL NUTRITION AND HYDRATION

A number of courts have addressed the issue of the right to withhold or withdraw artificial hydration or nutrition. Both the American Medical Association and American Nurses Association have issued statements supporting this patient right.

As discussed by the American Medical Association in its "Statement on Withholding or Withdrawing Life-Prolonging Medical Treatment," when a patient loses the ability to swallow because of the disease process, insertion of a feeding tube or IV is a medical treatment to resist the effects of the disease and to prolong life artificially. Consequently, there is no difference between this type of medical treatment and any other forms of treatment.

The American Nurses Association Committee on Ethics issued its "Guidelines on Withdrawing or Withholding Food and Fluid." An aspect of nursing care is the provision of food and fluid, and under most circumstances it is not morally permissible to withhold or withdraw these. It is, however, morally permissible when a patient is clearly more harmed by receiving food or fluid than by withholding them. For example, a patient preparing for or just recovering from surgery, infants with a tracheo-esophageal fistula or anal atresia, or patients with certain overeating disorders are certainly going to be more harmed by being fed than by withholding food. Yet, only these circumstances are normally temporary, and justify limited withholding.

The ANA Guidelines emphasize the importance of understanding a patient's reason for exercising the right to refuse hydration or nutrition. Verify that the patient understands the effects of withholding these. The refusal to accept food or fluid is not in and of itself evidence of incapacity. But a patient with the capacity to make a decision can refuse food or fluid because of inac-

---

32 *Id.* at 669.

curate facts or despair for reasons that are reversible. In those instances, a nurse should seek intervention on behalf of the patient who is exercising a right for the wrong reasons.

The American Dietetic Association has issued a Position Statement on feeding the terminally ill adult, with seven general standards regarding nutrition care for the terminally ill adult:

1. Each case is unique and must be handled individually.
2. The patient's expressed desire for the extent of medical care is a primary guide for determining the level of nutrition intervention.
3. The expected benefits, in contrast to the potential burdens, of non-oral feeding must be evaluated by the health care team and discussed with the patient. The focus of care should emphasize patient physical and psychological comfort.
4. The decision to forego hydration or nutrition support should be weighed carefully because such a decision may be difficult or impossible to reverse within a period of days or weeks.
5. The decision to forego "heroic" medical treatment does not preclude baseline nutrition support.
6. The physician's written diet order in the medical chart documents the decision to administer or forego nutrition support. The dietician should participate in this decision.
7. The institution's ethics committee, if available, should assist in establishing and implementing defined, written guidelines for nutrition support protocol. The dietician should be a required member of or consultant to such a committee.

In considering the efficacy of providing aggressive nutrition support, the following should be considered:

1. Will nutrient support, either oral or mechanical, improve the patient's quality of life during the final stages of morbidity by increasing physical strength or resistance to infections?
2. Will nutrient support, either oral or mechanical, provide the following to the patient: emotional comfort, decreased anxiety about disease, cachexia, improved self-esteem with cosmetic benefits, improved interpersonal relationships, or relief from the fear of abandonment?
3. Oral feedings are the preferred choice. Tube feeding is generally the next logical step. Parenteral nutrition should be considered only when other routes are impossible or inadequate to meet the comfort needs of the patient.

4. Oral intake

   a. Oral feedings should be advocated whenever possible. Food and control of food intake may give comfort and pleasure. The most important priority is to provide food according to the patient's individual wishes.

   b. Efforts should be made to enhance the patient's physical and emotional enjoyment of food by encouraging staff and family assistance in feeding the debilitated patient.

   c. Nutrition supplements, including commercial products and other alternatives, should be used to encourage intake and ameliorate symptoms associated with hunger, thirst, or malnutrition.

   d. The therapeutic rationale of previous diet prescriptions for an individual patient should be re-evaluated. Many dietary restrictions can be liberalized. Coordination of medication or medication schedules with the diet should be discussed with the physician, with the objective of maximizing food choice and intake by the patient.

   e. The patient's right to self-determination must be considered in determining whether to allow the patient to consume foods that are not generally permitted within the diet prescription.

5. Tube feeding or parenteral feeding

   a. Palliative care is a usual realistic goal. However, a palliative care plan does not automatically preclude aggressive nutrition support.

   b. Facilities should provide and distribute written protocols for the provision of and termination of tube feedings and parenteral feedings. The protocols should be reviewed periodically and revised if necessary by the health care team. Legal and ethical counsel should be routinely sought during the development and interpretation of the guidelines.

   c. The patient's informed preference for the level of nutrition intervention is paramount. The patient or guardian should be advised on how to accomplish feeding if the patient wanted maximal nutrition care.

   d. Feeding may not be desirable if death is expected within hours or a few days and the effects of partial dehydration or the withdrawal of nutrition support will not adversely alter patient comfort.

e. Potential benefits versus burdens of tube feeding or parenteral feeding should be weighed on the basis of specific facts concerning the patient's medical and mental status, as well as on facility options and limitations.[33]

A significant case regarding the rights of an individual to withhold or withdraw nutrition or hydration is *Cruzan v. Director, Missouri Department of Health*.[34] Nancy Beth Cruzan was rendered incompetent as a result of severe injuries sustained during an automobile accident. Nancy's parents, who were her legally appointed guardians, sought a court order directing the withdrawal of Nancy's artificial feeding and hydration equipment after it became apparent that she had no chance of recovering her cognitive faculties. At the time of the initial request to withdraw Nancy's feeding tube, she had been in a persistent vegetative state for over four years. Medical experts testified that she could live another thirty years if provided artificial nutrition and hydration.

Nancy's parents sought and received authorization from the Missouri trial court to terminate of the artificial nutrition and hydration procedures. That decision was appealed to the Missouri Supreme Court, and ultimately appealed to the United States Supreme Court.

The United States Supreme Court noted that "bodily integrity" has been embodied in the requirement that informed consent be obtained before providing medical treatment, and that the logical corollary of the doctrine of informed consent is that the patient generally possesses the right *not* to consent, that is, to refuse treatment. The Supreme Court also accepted as fact that there is no difference between treatment by artificial feeding versus other forms of life-sustaining medical procedures, nor is there any distinction between ordinary versus extraordinary treatment. Feeding by implanted tubes is a medical procedure with inherent risks and possible side effects, instituted to compensate for impaired physical functioning, which is analytically equivalent to artificial breathing using a respirator.

The Supreme Court however upheld the right of the Missouri Supreme Court to require clear and convincing evidence of what an individual wants before life-sustaining treatment is withheld or withdrawn. To establish this level of evidence, the Supreme Court advocated the use of advance directives and surrogate decision-makers. In passing, the Supreme Court also noted that family members have no constitutional right to act for an individual; States must specifically authorize family members as the decision-makers for patients.

---

33 The American Dietetic Association. *Position of The American Dietetic Association: Issues in Feeding the Terminally Ill Adult*, 92 Journal of the American Dietetic Association 995 (August 1992).

34 497 U.S. 261, 111 L. Ed. 2d 224, 110 S. Ct. 2841 (1990).

Following the decision of the United States Supreme Court, in November 1990, Nancy's parents again sought an order authorizing the removal of the artificial procedures providing nutrition and hydration to Nancy. The Missouri trial court found clear and convincing evidence that Nancy, if mentally able, would desire to terminate her nutrition and hydration in light of her present existence and slowly progressively worsening. It is important to note that the Judge found clear and convincing evidence through testimony of family and friends because Nancy had not left any advance directives.

In 2001, a court had the opportunity to apply the clear and convincing evidence standard that was legitimated by *Cruzan*. In *Conservatorship of Wendland*[35], the California Supreme Court considered a case involving the conservator of a patient, who sought to remove the patient's artificial nutrition and hydration. The patient suffered from severe brain damage due to a car accident. Although the patient was severely disabled, both physically and mentally, he was conscious and had limited abilities to communicate. The conservator proffered, as clear and convincing evidence, two informal pre-accident statements made by the patient, in which he expressed his desire never to live like a "vegetable." The California Supreme Court upheld the ruling of the trial court, which had articulated that:

> these two conversations do not establish by clear and convincing evidence that the conservatee would desire to have his life-sustaining medical treatment terminated under the circumstances in which he now finds himself. . . . The court finds that neither of these conversations reflect an exact "on all-fours" description of the conservatee's present medical condition. More explicit direction than just "I don't want to live like a vegetable" is required in order to justify a surrogate decision-maker terminating the life of someone who is not in a persistent vegetative state.[36]

The Court, therefore, denied the conservator's request to withdraw artificial nutrition and hydration from the patient.

SECTION 8-9: ASSISTED SUICIDE

Assisted suicide occurs when a physician or other care provider facilitates a patient's death by providing the required medications or information to enable the patient to perform a life-ending act. To fall within the definition of physician-assisted suicide (PAS), the patient himself must perform the suicidal act.

PAS is often confused with active euthanasia. According to the American Medical Association Code of Ethics standard E-2.21, euthanasia "is the admin-

---

35   28 P.3d 151 (Cal. 2001).

36   *Id.* at 173.

istration of a lethal agent by another person to a patient for the purpose of relieving the patient's intolerable and incurable suffering." To fall within the definition of euthanasia, it is the care giver who must perform the life-ending act. Euthanasia is illegal in every state in the United States, and is not supported by the American Medical Association nor the American Nurses Association. The remainder of the discussion in this section will focus solely on PAS.

PAS is illegal in every state except Oregon. Some states criminalize PAS by classifying it as a homicide, manslaughter, or some other homicide crime. Many states have now enacted statutes that explicitly outlaw PAS.

The American Medical Association, in its Code of Ethics Standard E-2.211, has declared PAS "fundamentally incompatible with the physician's role as healer." Similarly, the American Nurses Association (ANA) believes that nurses should not participate in PAS. In a position statement, the ANA declared that, while nurses must provide relief of suffering in a manner that is consistent with the wishes of a dying patient, nurses should uphold the ethical values of the nursing profession and should not participate in assisted suicide.

In 1997, two important United States Supreme Court decisions were rendered that involve PAS. *Washington v. Glucksberg*[37], involved three terminally ill patients, four physicians and a nonprofit organization who challenged a Washington state law that made promoting a suicide a felony. The plaintiffs argued that the liberty interest guaranteed by the Fourteenth Amendment's Due Process Clause extended to the personal choice of a mentally competent, terminally ill adult to commit PAS.

The United States Supreme Court, however, upheld the validity of the Washington law by ruling that the law did not violate the Due Process Clause of the Fourteenth Amendment.[38] The Supreme Court reasoned that Washington's ban on assisted suicide was closely related to the following state interests:

1. Preserving human life and preventing suicide;
2. Protecting the integrity and ethics of the medical profession;
3. Protecting vulnerable groups, such as the poor, elderly and disabled; and
4. Avoiding the slippery slope to state approval of voluntary or involuntary euthanasia.

In a companion case, *Vacco v. Quill*[39], the United States Supreme Court considered the validity of a New York statute that made it a crime to aid a per-

---

37 521 U.S. 702 (1997).

38 *Id.* at 702.

39 521 U.S. 793.

son to commit suicide or to attempt to commit suicide. Plaintiffs in this case based their challenge on the Equal Protection Clause of the Fourteenth Amendment, which demands that state laws provide the same protections to classes of similarly situated individuals. Plaintiffs argued that the distinction between refusing lifesaving medical treatment, which was legal in New York, and assisted suicide, which was outlawed by the statute, was arbitrary and irrational. The Supreme Court, however, ruled that the State ban on assisted suicide did not violate the Equal Protection Clause, and upheld the validity of the New York law.[40] When read together, these cases indicate that there is no constitutionally protected right to PAS, but that States may individually decide to legalize or otherwise regulate PAS.

To date, Oregon is the only State that has legalized PAS. In 1997, Oregon voters approved the Oregon Death with Dignity Act for the second time, after a prior referendum vote was challenged in court. To commit PAS under the Act, a patient must be an adult resident of Oregon, whose terminal illness will cause death within six months, and who makes a voluntary, written request to end his life. The Act contains a number of safeguards designed to prevent inappropriate instances of PAS. First, the Act requires that a patient be diagnosed as terminally ill by both his attending and a consulting physician. Second, the Act requires that patients who suffer from psychiatric disorders or depression be referred for counseling. Third, the Act requires an extensive informed consent process prior to the PAS, which demands disclosure to the patient of his diagnosis, prognosis, and feasible alternatives to PAS such as hospice and palliative care. Finally, the statute requires a fifteen day waiting period between the request for PAS and carrying out the act.

Oregon publishes an annual report on the Death with Dignity Act that summarizes PAS statistics under the Act. In 2002, fifty-eight prescriptions were written under the Act to patients who desired to end their lives. Of those prescriptions that were written, only thirty-eight recipients ingested the medication and ended their lives. In the five years, from 1997 until 2002, that PAS has been legal in Oregon, one hundred and twenty-nine individuals have committed PAS under the Act. The Fifth Annual Report on Oregon's Death with Dignity Act notes that the majority of individuals who committed PAS were older (the average age was sixty-nine years), well educated, and had cancer. Due to widespread constituency disapproval of PAS and the possibility that more states will legalize PAS, Congress in 1997 passed the Assisted Suicide Funding Restriction Act, which disallows federal financial assistance in support of PAS.[41] The Act contains a Congressional finding that "Assisted suicide, euthanasia, and mercy killing have been criminal offenses through the United

---

40 *Id.* at 796.

41 42 U.S.C. § 14401.

States and, under current law, it would be unlawful to provide services in support of such illegal activities."[42]

PAS jurisprudence also contains important implications for pain management in terminally-ill patients. PAS should not be confused with palliative treatment that has the incidental effect of hastening a patient's death.

The principle of double effect holds that each inherently good action has two effects: (1) the intended good effect (i.e. to relieve pain); and (2) an unintended, yet foreseeable bad effect (i.e. to hasten death by prescribing pain medications that depress respiration). The principle demands that the benefit of the good effect be greater than the foreseeable bad effects. Care givers need not abstain from a good action that has foreseeable bad effects. Under this principle, most care providers agree that it is ethically permissible to increase pain medication to a patient with the knowledge that the medication may depress respiration and lead to the death of the patient.

In her concurring opinion to *Glucksberg* and *Quill*, Justice O'Connor indicated that there is a constitutionally protected right to medications to manage pain:

> In sum, there is no need to address the question whether suffering patients have a constitutionally cognizable interest in obtaining relief from the suffering that they may experience in the last days of their lives. There is no dispute that dying patients in Washington and New York can obtain palliative care even when doing so would hasten their deaths.[43]

REFERENCES

American Academy of Neurology, *Practice Parameters: Assessment and Management of Patients in the Persistent Vegetative State (Summary Statement)*. The Quality Standards Subcommittee of the American Academy of Neurology, 45 Neurology 1015 (May 1995).

American Academy of Pediatrics, Committee on Bioethics. *Guidelines on Forgoing Life-Sustaining Medical Treatment*, 93 Pediatrics 532 (March 1994).

American Medical Association's Council on Ethical and Judicial Affairs, *Withholding or Withdrawing Life-Prolonging Medical Treatment* (June 1966).

---

42 *Id.*

43 *Glucksberg, supra*, at 738.

American Nurses Association Task Force on End of Life Decisions, *Position Statement on Forgoing Artificial Nutrition and Hydration,* (1992).

American Nurses Association, *Code of Ethics for Nurses with Interpretive Statements* (2001), at http://www.nursingworld.org/ethics/code/ethicscode150.htm.

American Society of PeriAnesthesia Nurses, *A Position Statement on the Perianesthesia Patient with a Do-not-Resuscitate Advance Directive,* (April 20, 1996).

American Thoracic Society, P*osition Paper: Withholding and Withdrawing Life-Sustaining Therapy*, 115 Annals of Internal Medicine 478 (Sept. 15, 1991).

Association of Operating Room Nurses, Inc, *Position Statement: Perioperative Care of Patients with Do-Not-Resuscitate* (DNR) Orders (October 1999).

Christopherson, R., *Suspension of DNR Orders During the Perioperative Period: The Johns Hopkins Policy*, Perspectives in Healthcare Risk Management 4 (Fall 1991).

Colby, W. H., *The Lessons of the Cruzan Case*, 39 The University of Kansas Law Review 519 (1991).

Council on Ethical and Judicial Affairs, American Medical Association, *Guidelines for the Appropriate Use of Do-Not-Resuscitate Orders.* 265 JAMA 1868 (Apr. 10, 1991).

Council on Scientific Affairs, American Medical Association, *Good Care of the Dying Patient,* 275 JAMA 474 (February 14, 1996).

Daar, Judith, F., *Medical Futility and Implications for Physician Autonomy,* 21 American Journal of Law & Medicine 221 (1995).

Drew, M., and Fleming, V. M. *The Nurse's Role in Supporting Patients' Treatment Decisions,* 2 Journal of Nursing Law 27 (1995).

Herlik, A., *Medicine at the Margins: Our National Struggle With Medically Futile Treatments*, 3 Journal of Nursing Law 63 (1996).

Joint Commission on Accreditation of Healthcare Organizations, *Comprehensive Accreditation Manual for Hospitals: The Official Handbook* (2004).

Mendelson, D., *Historical Evolution and Modern Implications of Concepts of Consent to and Refusal of Medical Treatment in the Law of Trespass,* 17 Journal of Legal Medicine 1 (1996).

President's Commission for the Study of Ethical Problems in Medicine and Biomedical and Behavioral Research, *Deciding to Forego Life-Sustaining Treatment,* No. 83-600503 (1983).

President's Commission for the Study of Ethical Problems in Medicine and Biomedical and Behavioral Research, *Making Health Care Decisions: The Ethical and Legal Implications of Informed Consent and the Patient-Practitioner Relationship,* No. 82-6000637 1-3 (1982).

Sabatino, C. P., *10 Legal Myths About Advance Medical Directives.* 3 Journal of Nursing Law 35 (1996).

Scanlon, Marybeth, *Providing Eid-of-Life Care in Connecticut: Should Nurses Fear Liability?* 5 Buinnipiac Health Law J. 35 (2001).

State of Oregon, Department of Human Services, *Fifth Annual Report on Oregon's Death with Dignity Act* (March 6, 2003).

The American College of Obstetricians and Gynecologists Committee on Ethics, *End-of-Life Decision Making: Understanding the Goals of Care* (May 1995).

The American Dietetic Association, *Position of the American Dietetic Association: Issues in Feeding the Terminally Ill Adult,* 92 Journal of the American Dietetic Association 995 (August 1992).

CHAPTER 9

Special Practice Areas

SECTION 9-1: ACUTE CARE/HOSPITAL

The Emergency Department is a high risk area with a large number of malpractice claims arising out of treatment rendered there. Patients seen in the Emergency Department are typically seriously ill or injured and therefore more likely to suffer a significant disability or death, which tends to promote litigation. The atmosphere in the Emergency Department may seem impersonal and rushed, and patients may have to wait for an extended period of time before being examined and treated. These negative perceptions adversely affect how patients feel they have been treated. Documentation by Emergency Department providers is typically incomplete because they neglect the necessary time to document comprehensively. In the Emergency Department, nurses and physicians aren't able to establish a strong relationship with a patient, much less a positive one.

If a surgeon attempts to perform a procedure beyond those specific procedures identified on the consent form, in the absence of an emergency or unforeseeable event, that violates the patient's right of consent. When a nurse becomes aware that a surgeon is adding procedures to an already executed consent, the nurse is responsible for reporting that physician through the appropriate channels. This constitutes falsification of a legal document and will result in performing an unauthorized procedure on the patient, which is a battery. The nurse's failure to appropriately intervene and report any such knowledge could be construed as a conspiracy between the nurse and surgeon to perpetrate a battery upon the patient.

Perioperative nurses need to have a list of those physicians who have staff privileges at the hospital or ambulatory surgical center and their privileges.

These are to be checked and any violations reported as set forth in the facility's procedures.

In the post-anesthesia area, it is important that clear lines of responsibility and authority for patient care decisions are delineated. Frequently these are absent, thereby placing the nurse in a position of not knowing what physician to call. Typically surgeons and anesthesiologists are at odds with one another or think the other is taking responsibility for the patient. For the benefit of the nurse and patient, responsibilities must be clarified and followed.

Equipment used in the perioperative area also creates potential liabilities. Nurses must be familiar with equipment they are responsible for using and must maintain their competency with that equipment. If a nurse is unfamiliar with a piece of equipment, it is the nurse's responsibility to put the appropriate nurse administrator on notice that adequate inservices are necessary prior to that equipment being used.

If a nurse observes equipment being used improperly by a physician, the nurse has a duty of affirmative action to act on the patient's behalf. In addition to alerting the physician that the equipment is not being used correctly, the nurse must take any necessary steps to correct the problem.

Frequent allegations in hospitals relate to restraints and falls. Margaret Thomas was 82 years old and lived independently when her family began to notice changes in her behavior, such as irrationality, forgetfulness, and an impaired sense of time. She was taken to University of Cinncinati Medical Center and diagnosed with dementia.[1] During the first 48 hours, Mrs. Thomas was polite and cooperative. However, two days after her admission, she attempted to get out of bed and slipped on urine that was present on the floor. As she slipped, a nurse grabbed her arm and prevented any injury. Mrs. Thomas then became agitated. The nurse calmed her, administered a prescribed sedative, and placed her in a geri-chair.

Later that morning, the nurses placed Mrs. Thomas back into her Hospital bed with the siderails up and instructed her not to get out of bed without assistance. She slept until noon. Upon awakening, Mrs. Thomas refused to eat lunch, but took her prescribed medication and again fell asleep. At approximately 3:00 p.m., Mrs. Thomas' daughter arrived for a visit. At that time, Mrs. Thomas was discovered to have allegedly fallen to the floor in her room.

Mrs. Thomas filed an action against the Hospital, alleging that the nurses deviated from the accepted standards of psychiatric nursing care in its monitoring of Mrs. Thomas by failing to implement one-on-one, continuous, in-room supervision of Mrs. Thomas. Mrs. Thomas also alleged that the Hospital was negligent in its failure to place Mrs. Thomas in some form of physical restraint.

---

1 *Barnette v. University of Cinncinati Hospital*, 702 N.E.2d 979 (Ohio App. 1998).

As a result of these deviations from the established standards of psychiatric nursing care, Mrs. Thomas fell and sustained a subdural hematoma.

At trial, Mrs. Thomas offered expert testimony as did the defendant Hospital. Based upon the expert testimony, the court concluded that the nurses *did not deviate* from the standard of care expected of them, but in fact exercised appropriate care by maintaining close supervision through periodic checks of Mrs. Thomas and by placing her in a room within eye sight of the nurses station. "Defendant's nurses used good judgment, made accurate assessments of Thomas' condition, and implemented reasonable, logical nursing care."[2] Accordingly, judgment was rendered in favor of University of Cinncinati Hospital.

A significant number of cases arise from allegations of failing to monitor and failing to timely notify physicians of significant changes in a patient's condition. This was the key issue in *Miller v. Heartland Regional Medical Center*.[3] Marianne Miller was injured in an auto accident as she was traveling to high school at 7 am on Friday, October 6, 1995. Marianne felt back pain right away and an ambulance was called to the scene. When the ambulance arrived, Marianne was able to move her toes, legs and feet, and had feeling in her toes, feet and legs.

At the Medical Center an x-ray was taken that confirmed a fractured vertebrae putting pressure on Marianne's spinal canal and interrupting the supply of blood and oxygen to the spinal cord. The attending neurosurgeon concluded that surgery was necessary to remove the offending bone. But because he was not qualified to perform a crucial part of the surgery, he decided to transfer the patient to another neurosurgeon. However, this neurosurgeon was on vacation and would not be available until the following week. The attending neurosurgeon decided to schedule the operation for several days later when his partner would return. He left instructions with the nurses to watch Marianne closely for signs for neurological worsening, and informed her family that he would perform emergency surgery if her condition deteriorated.

The neurosurgeon specifically ordered the nurses to test Marianne's neurological function on an hourly basis and inform him of any changes. But although the medical records kept by the nurses reflected the steady worsening of Marianne's neurological function over the weekend, the nurses failed to recognize the significance and did not inform the neurosurgeon. On the evening of her admission, Marianne could not longer wiggle her toes; by the next morning, she could no longer lift her legs.

---

2 *Id.* at 981.

3 *Miller v. Heartland Regional Medical Center*, Case No.: CV396-1770cc (Buchanan County Circuit Court 1998).

According to the nurses, they failed to realize the changes occurring in Marianne's condition because they were unaware of what her condition was when she was admitted. When the nurse noted that Marianne couldn't wiggle her toes, she thought Marianne could never wiggle her toes and so didn't recognize it as a change. However, it was noted that on the same page of the medical record on which the nurse documented it was clearly written that Marianne *could* wiggle her toes earlier in the day.

Another issue was the lack of a systematic method for evaluating Marianne's neurological function. Instead of testing the strength of her muscles and recording numerical scores for each muscle group, they documented their observations in vague terms. At trial, two representatives of the Medical Center gave contradictory testimony to questions about the lack of a system of measurement and reporting of neurological function. One corporate designee said the nurses were taught the systematic test as the way to record neurological functioning scores. Another supervising nurse said there's "no standard" for how it is supposed to be done so each nurse does it in her own way.

There was also conflicting testimony about what the nurses were required to report to the neurosurgeon. According to the neurosurgeon, he left clear instructions that the nurses were to inform him of "any" change, while the nurses felt they were supposed to report any changes that were "important."

The nurses were documenting "medical conclusions," such as phrases like "neuros unchanged," rather than raw data. Thus, when the neurosurgeon saw Marianne on Saturday, he concluded, in large part based upon the nursing documentation, that her condition was unchanged. It wasn't until Sunday, October 8 that the neurosurgeon first noticed that Marianne had lost strength in her legs and realized for the first time that her condition had worsened. There was then a delay to perform the surgery; it wasn't performed until the afternoon of October 9. Prior to trial, Marianne settled with the neurosurgeon for an undisclosed amount of money.

The jury concluded that the Medical Center was negligent and apportioned 50% of the fault to the Medical Center because of the nurses' negligence. The verdict was $2.75 million, including $1 million in non-economic damages.

The *common knowledge* doctrine, also known as *res ipsa loquitor*, was found to apply when a patient died during a hysteroscopy, a diagnostic procedure in which death is not an anticipated risk.[4] During the procedure, a Bard Hystero-Flo Pump was used, which is a device consisting of several tubes and a pump. Fluid is inserted into the uterus via the pump which is energized by nitrogen gas. Gas that has powered the pump flows out of the system through an open

---

4 *Chin v. St. Barnabas Medical Center*, 711 A.2d 352 (N.J. App. 1998), *aff'd*, 734 A.2d 778 (N.J. 1999).

exhaust line into the atmosphere. Excess fluid is evacuated from the uterus through a suction tube attached to the outflow port. Sometimes gravity is used to evacuate the fluid, or a section canister facilitates evacuation. During the diagnostic procedure on Angela Chin, gas entered through her body cavity and into her circulatory system. Air bubbles formed in her blood vessels and killed her almost immediately. All parties agree that the exhaust line was the source of the gas that killed Mrs. Chin.

There was complicated testimony about the pump, the different lines and clips used to keep the exhaust lines and suction lines in place. The result was that no one clearly knew what happened, how it happened, or why it happened.

The court noted that numerous conclusions could be reached by the jury. One of the nurses could have removed a clip or caused it to come off the exhaust line. Dr. Goldfarb could have attached the loose exhaust line to the outflow port. The exhaust line could have been unclipped, inadvertently or purposefully, that made it possible for that line to be within the operative field, thereby facilitating its erroneous connection to the outflow port. Or one of the nurses could have connected the loose exhaust line to a suction canister which may have been connected to the scope through the suction tubing.

It was clear that the two nurses assisting in the procedure had no experiencing using this Bard pump as they had not attended the Medical Center training sessions. The supervising nurse who made the assignments was unaware of their lack of experience. Because of their experience, the two assigned nurses then asked another nurse to assist them.

The court concluded that "reason and common sense dictate that . . . under the peculiar circumstances of this case the occurrence itself indicates liability on the part of one or more of the defendants, and that the burden should be shifted to defendants as they are most likely to possess knowledge of the cause of the accident."[5] When it is apparent that at least one of the defendants is liable for a patient's injury because no alternative theory of liability is reasonably contemplated, the failure of any defendant to prove nonculpability triggers liability. This shifts the burden of proof to the defendants.

SECTION 9-2: ADVANCED PRACTICE

The standard of care for nurses in advanced practice will generally be higher than the standard of care for the basic-level registered nurse. The standard is generally the same as the standard of care for a physician for activities that may be performed by either a nurse or physician.

---

5 *Id.* at 355.

195

In States that do not specifically define advanced practice, it is imperative for nurses who are functioning in expanded roles to make certain that they have the authority to function pursuant to their State's Nurse Practice Act. Some Nurse Practice Acts are written broadly enough to encompass advanced practice.

Many States, through statutes or regulations, define advanced practice and the requirements necessary to gain and use that title. These may include requirements that nurses in advanced practice function pursuant to written protocols. Protocols are written documents that are developed in collaboration with and approved by a physician. They establish guidelines for nurses to independently diagnose and treat patients, including dispensing and perhaps prescribing medications. Protocols are different from standing orders in that standing orders *mandate* what nurses must do while protocols allow nurses to *exercise their judgment* as to when and how the protocols should be implemented.

The types of potential claims that may be brought against nurses in advanced practice will generally be the same ones that are brought against other nurses. However, nurses in advanced practice may have increased potential for liability because they more frequently make independent professional judgments, have greater responsibilities for patient management, and directly impact patient outcomes.

The administrator of the estate of a patient who died from breast cancer brought a wrongful death action against two physicians and a nurse practitioner based on alleged failure to diagnose cancer.[6] Veronica Payne first sought treatment for breast abnormalities on January 7, 1991. She was examined by Jill York, a nurse practitioner working under the supervision of Dr. Jenkins. Ms. Payne informed Nurse York that, for a period of seven months, she had been experiencing a discharge and constant scabbing of her left nipple. Nurse York ordered a mammogram and prescribed oral and topical antibiotics as treatment for infection of the nipple. The mammogram showed no signs of tumors in the breast.

On July 18, 1991, Ms. Payne returned to Nurse York complaining of the continuing pain and discharge from her left breast. Nurse York referred her to a dermatologist for treatment of the continuing irritation. Nurse York testified that she believed the dermatologist would perform a biopsy of the abnormal tissue.

The medical records reflect that Nurse York didn't discussed with Ms. Payne the need for a biopsy or the possibility of cancer. Nurse York testified that she did not determine whether Ms. Payne followed up with the dermatologist or the result of that examination.

---

6 *Jenkins v. Payne*, 465 S.E.2d 795 (Va. 1996).

On October 21, 1991, and November 8, 1991, Ms. Payne sought treatment from Dr. Rothman, a gynecologist. Dr. Rothman recorded Ms. Payne's history that, for a period of one and one-half years, she had suffered from an inflamed and bleeding left nipple. Dr. Rothman prescribed oral antibiotics and a topical steroid cream to treat the condition. Ms. Payne expressed relief to Dr. Rothman that he had reassured her she was only suffering from eczema; she was afraid she had cancer.

Ms. Payne made visits to Nurse York on January 29, February 27, and March 12, 1992. Ms. Payne's medical records indicate that she was concerned about "sores that have been slow to heal." Nurse York testified that she could not recall whether she had discussed with Ms. Payne any problems about her breast. Ms. Payne's medical records reflect that neither Nurse York or Dr. Jenkins made any other examination of Ms. Payne's breast or that they pursued their recommendation that she to see a specialist.

On September 23, 1992, Nurse York examined Ms. Payne and discovered the presence of multiple masses in Ms. Payne's breast. In December 1992, Ms. Payne began receiving treatment from a surgical oncologist, Dr. Wilhelm. He determined that the cancer had spread to her lymph nodes and was particularly aggressive, rendering her prognosis poor and the terminal nature of the cancer certain. In December 1992, Ms. Payne was diagnosed with Paget's disease in its terminal stage. At that time, she had palpable masses in her left breast and had been experiencing continual soreness and discharge from her left nipple for two years. She died in April 1994.

The evidence at trial showed that Paget's disease is a cancer of the nipple and milk ducts. Abnormalities of the nipple, including discharge and lesions, are classic symptoms of the disease. In the early stages, no mass is present in the breast tissue. Thus, mammography does not indicate the presence of the cancer in its early stages, and a biopsy is the best method of providing a timely diagnosis. Paget's disease is not invasive in its early stages, grows slowly, and is highly curable. It can remain non-invasive for several years. There is about a 90% survival rate for patients with Paget's Disease who receive treatment before the cancer becomes invasive.

At trial, Dr. Wilhelm testified that Ms. Payne would have had a ten-year survival probability of nearly 90% if her cancer had been diagnosed when it was still non-invasive. Dr. Neifeld, a surgical oncologist, stated that Ms. Payne's cancer became invasive three to six months prior to her December 1992 diagnosis.

Dr. Mackintosh, an expert in primary care medicine, testified that the standard of care for treatment of the breast is the same for a family practice physician and nurse practitioner as for a gynecologist. Dr. Mackintosh and Dr. Neifeld both testified that, beginning in January 1991, Nurse York and Dr. Jenkins breached the standard of care by failing to recognize symptoms of breast cancer, by overemphasizing the possibility of infection rather than cancer, by failing to refer Ms. Payne to a surgeon for biopsy, and by failing to determine whether the surgeon had diagnosed the breast abnormality. They testified that Nurse York and Dr. Jenkins breached the standard of care on Ms. Payne's 1991 visits as well as on her January, February and March 1992 visits.

Yvonne Newberry, an expert on the standard of care for family nurse practitioners, testified that given Ms. Payne's history of breast problems, Nurse York should have performed a breast examination and discussed the possibility of cancer with Ms. Payne during the January, February and March 1992 office visits. Nurse Newberry testified that Nurse York had an obligation to ask Ms. Payne about the status of the breast even when Ms. Payne did not specifically complain about it.

Margaret Light, a nurse practitioner, testified that Nurse York met the standard of care in ordering a mammogram, suggesting a conservative plan of treatment with antibiotics, and instructing Ms. Payne on what action she should take if her symptoms did not improve. Dr. Muller, an expert in primary care medicine, testified that Nurse York and Dr. Jenkins met the standard of care by treating Ms. Payne to the best of their ability and by referring her to a dermatologist for additional care. Dr. Muller stated that Ms. Payne then bore the responsibility to follow their advice and to consult a specialist.

Based on all of the testimony that was presented at trial, the jury determined that both Nurse York and Dr. Jenkins failed to meet the standard of care and their failure resulted in the death of Ms. Payne. The jury returned a verdict awarding $1.1 million in damages to the estate of Ms. Payne. Prior to trial, the gynecologist had settled his claim for $450,000.

Malpractice litigation for nurse midwives is not common. However, these nurses are certainly not exempt from being sued. This was evident by a case that was settled on behalf of a six-year-old child who has spastic quadriplegia, no sphincter control, is unable to speak, but has an approximately normal intellect.[7]

The mother, a 28-year-old actress, chose home delivery because she was extremely adverse to having her baby in a hospital. Her obstetrical care was provided by two certified nurse midwives who were partners. They were very experienced, having managed about 800 home births, and had never been sued for malpractice. They had an obstetrician available as a back up, both for telephone consultation and delivery.

At 6:00 a.m. on June 27, the mother's membranes ruptured. She telephoned the first nurse midwife, who arrived quickly, and observed an amniotic-fluid soaked towel that revealed light meconium staining. At 7:30 a.m., the cervix was

---

7 *A Two Million-Plus Settlement by Two Nurse Midwives*, 24 Professional Liability Newsletter 1 (December 1993).

dilated 2–3 centimeters, and in the afternoon dilation was 8–9 centimeters. There was then a marginal delay in the progress of labor.

About an hour and a half before birth, the second midwife was called. According to the first midwife, she had trouble in reducing an anterior cervical lip, and she knew her partner was more skillful at handling such a problem. She also felt her partner might be more persuasive if the mother had to be convinced to go to the hospital. After the second midwife arrived, there was no further difficulty until the baby crowned at 6:00 p.m. A shoulder dystocia was recognized, but the usual maneuvers to overcome the dystocia were ineffective. It was then five of six minutes before a deep episiotomy was done; it then took less than a minute to accomplish delivery. At birth the baby was profoundly cyanotic. The Apgar scores at both one and five minutes were 2. The heart rate was 100.

During delivery there was discharge of a large amount of meconium, and it was apparent the infant had aspirated some. An aspirator was used and meconium was obtained, but the nurses did not have an endotracheal tube. Although they were trained in its use, they did not believe they could maintain the skill to perform intubation without error. They had an oxygen tank at the bedside and immediately administered oxygen with an Ambu bag. But the tank would only produce four liters a minute rather than the usual six liters. A second tank was obtained from the car, which yielded a normal flow.

The paramedics were not called until five to seven minutes after delivery. The reason offered for the delay was that "sometimes babies pink up." The paramedics arrived about four minutes after they had been contacted and transported the baby to a hospital. One of the midwives rode in the ambulance with the baby and she testified that she repeatedly asked the paramedic to administer oxygen, but he only used the Ambu bag on room air.

The emergency medicine physician immediately intubated the baby and suctioned her, but he did not aspirate all of the meconium, as proven when more meconium was obtained after the infant was transferred to a children's hospital. However, there was some delay before the baby was transferred.

Had the case been tried, a significant issue for the nurse midwives were the failure to quickly perform a deep episiotomy as soon as the shoulder dystocia was recognized, and the inability to accomplish endotracheal intubation. There was also the poor performance of the first oxygen tank and the delay in calling the paramedics. Another issue was whether because of the meconium stained amniotic fluid and the rather slow dilatation, the nurse midwives should have identified this as a greater than normal risk of labor and therefore transported the patient to the hospital. It seemed clear that there was a degree of reluctance by the nurse midwives to regard this as an other than normal labor because of the mother's fear of hospitalization.

It was the plaintiff's position that the nurse midwives, having decided not to transfer the mother to the hospital where the back-up obstetrician was readily available, had to perform as well as an obstetrician under similar circumstances. It was noted that there has been no appellate decision in California on this particular question. However, in another case, a notary public who negligently wrote a will, causing financial loss to the intended heirs, was held to the same standard as a probate attorney. Certainly nurse midwives are held to the same standards as obstetricians in other aspects of obstetrical care and treatment.

This case was settled with the insurance carrier for the two nurse midwives contributing $2.1 million to the settlement. $230,000 was paid on behalf of the paramedics and emergency medical physician.

The liability of a surgeon for the actions of a CRNA was the issue here. Sharilynn Starcher was admitted to Golf Coast Medical Center for elective surgery to correct a ventral hernia which was performed by Dr. Byrne.[8] CRNA William Wright was responsible for the anesthesia. At the beginning of the anesthesia induction, Dr. Byrne received an emergency page concerning another patient so went into the hallway to answer the page. After completing the telephone call, Dr. Byrne returned to the operating room where he noticed that there was problem with the anesthesia induction. Dr. Byrne and CRNA Wright determined that Sharilynn was suffering from a bronchospasm. Emergency treatment was provided and CPR was successfully administered. However, as a result of her inability to breath and the failure of her heart to pump blood to her brain for several minutes, Sharilynn suffered brain damage resulting in decreased intellectual and physical capacity. The patient and her husband filed the action against Dr. Byrne alleging that he was negligent for not being present in the operating room at the induction of anesthesia.

The weight of the expert witness testimony established there was no requirement for a physician to be physically present in the operating room at the induction of anesthesia. The common practice is for the surgeon to be in the operating suite, which is consistent with the Medical Center's policy. There was also sufficient evidence that CRNA Wright could administer anesthesia where neither a surgeon nor an anesthesiologist is present in the operating room. In Mississippi, CRNAs are licensed to do so and this is a common practice.

The plaintiffs argued that Dr. Byrne is liable as a matter of law for the conduct of CRNA Wright under the borrowed servant rule. Yet there were not cases cited holding that a CRNA, or any other nurse for that matter, is a borrowed servant of the operating surgeon during the course of surgery. IN determining whether the borrowed servant relationship is applicable, consider these three

---

8 *Starcher v. Byrne*, 687 S.2d 737 (Miss. 1997).

important factors: (1) whose work is being performed; (2) did Dr. Byrne have the right to control CRNA Wright in his duties; and (3) was there an employment contract either actual or implied between CRNA Wright and Dr. Byrne.

In this case, the court concluded that Dr. Byrne had no right of control over CRNA Wright, nor was CRNA Wright under any obligation to obey the orders of Dr. Byrne. CRNA Wright was never under the direction and control of Dr. Byrne and no special contract of employment existed between them. Thus, the court affirmed the jury verdict for Dr. Byrne.

SECTION 9-3: BEHAVIORAL HEALTH

The most significant case for mental health professionals remains the decision of the California Supreme Court in *Tarasoff v. Regents of the University of California*[9]. This was an action brought against a psychologist to recover for the murder of the plaintiff's daughter. Poddar, a patient of the psychologist, killed Tatiana Tarasoff two months after he had confided to the psychologist his intent to kill her. No one warned Tatiana about this threat against her. The plaintiff's action was based upon the psychologist's failure to warn of the impending danger.

In this decision, the court took note that the relationship of a physician to a patient is sufficient to support the duty to exercise reasonable care to protect others against dangers emanating from the patient's illness. Other courts have found physicians liable to persons infected by the physician's patient where there was a failure to diagnose a contagious disease or, having diagnosed the illness, failure to warn members of the patient's family. The court concluded that the role of the psychologist is like that of the physician who must conform to the standards of the profession and who must often make diagnoses and predictions based upon such evaluations. Thus, the judgment of the therapist in diagnosing emotional disorders and in predicting whether a patient presents a serious danger of violence is comparable to the judgment which physicians and professionals must regularly render under accepted rules of responsibility. As the court concluded:

> While the discharge of this duty of due care will necessarily vary with the facts of each case, in each instance the adequacy of the therapist's conduct must be measured against the traditional negligence standard of the rendition of reasonable care under the circumstances.[10]

Subsequent to *Tarasoff*, the court in *Thompson v. County of Alameda*[11], clarified its position by explaining that the duty recognized in *Tarasoff* does not

---

9 551 P.2d 334 (Cal. 1976).

10 *Id.* at 345.

11 614 P.2d 728 (Cal. 1980).

apply to the general public, but only arises when the intended victim is foreseeable and readily identifiable.[12] No affirmative duty to warn exists when a patient has made "non-specific threats of harm directed at non-specific victims."[13]

A *Tarasoff*-duty has been adopted in at least twenty-five states, either as a result of judicial decision, legislation, or both. Additional states have indicated that they would impose a duty to warn under facts similar to those present in *Tarasoff*. Only one court has expressly rejected the holding of *Tarasoff*.[14] Subsequent to this decision, Florida adopted legislation that permissibly allows a psychiatrist to disclose patient communications to the extent necessary to warn potential victims or law enforcement authorities.[15]

Missouri is one of the states that recently adopted the duty to warn as set forth in *Tarasoff*. In *Bradley v. Ray*[16], the court was asked to determine whether there is a common law duty to warn. The facts in this case are that Kelly Pope was allegedly abused by her stepfather, Lester Pope, from 1980, when she was four years old, until 1989. Kelly's mother, Nancy Kopin, became aware of the abuse and arranged to have Dr. Ray and Dr. Strnad render psychiatric services to Mr. Pope. Drs. Ray and Strnad were licensed psychologists with a practice in Columbia, Missouri. They began counseling Mr. Pope in 1988 for the abuse of Kelly but shortly thereafter terminated the counseling. It was alleged that Drs. Ray and Strnad were aware that Mr. Pope was abusing Kelly but failed to warn anyone of the abuse, including reporting as required under the Missouri Child Abuse Reporting Act.

In analyzing whether Missouri would recognize this theory of liability, the court focused on the principles commonly relied upon by other states in imposing a duty to warn. They include the foreseeability of the harm, the special relationship between the psychotherapist and patient, and the public policy of the state to discourage or prevent foreseeable harm. They also noted that consideration must be given to the magnitude of the burden to the practitioner of guarding against the injury and the consequences of placing that burden on the practitioner.

As in most states, the general rule under Missouri common law is "that a private person has no duty to protect another from deliberate criminal acts by a third person."[17] An exception arises if there is a special relationship between the parties that establishes a duty to control. A duty has been imposed on other med-

---

12 *Id.* at 734.

13 *Id.* at 735.

14 *Boynton v. Burglass*, 590 So.2d 446 (Fla. App. 1991).

15 Fla. Stat. Ann. § 455.2415 (West 1996).

16 904 S.W.2d 302 (Mo. App. 1995).

17 *Id.* at 311.

ical professionals, such as warning of communicable diseases that may be acquired by a third party. As the court concluded, "There is no reason why a similar duty to warn should not exist when the 'disease' of the patient is a mental illness that poses an analogous risk of harm to others."[18] However, this duty only arises where there is a foreseeable likelihood that particular acts or omissions will cause the harm or injury.[19]

The court held as follows:

> We hold that the public policy of this State, in addition to the special relationship between defendants and their patient, and the foreseeability of harm to Kelly, give rise to a duty on the part of defendants to warn appropriate authorities of the risk of future harm of Kelly by Mr. Pope. Specifically, we hold that when a psychologist or other health care professional knows or pursuant to the standards of his profession should have known that a patient presents a serious danger of future violence to a readily identifiable victim the psychologist has a duty under Missouri common law to warn the intended victim or communicate the existence of such danger to those likely to warn the victim including notifying appropriate enforcement authorities.[20]

A prevalent concern in health care is whether patients, especially those with behavioral health diagnoses, will be discharged inappropriately due to lack of health insurance. This was the precise issue presented to the jury in *Muse v. Charter Hospital of Winston-Salem, Inc.*[21] The parents of a child who committed suicide shortly after being discharged from the hospital brought a wrongful death action against the treating physician, hospital, and hospital corporation.

On June 12, 1986, Joe Muse, who was sixteen years old at the time, was admitted to Charter Hospital for treatment related to his depression and suicidal thoughts. Joe's treatment team consisted of Dr. Barnhill, Fernando Garzon, the nursing therapist, and Betsey Willard, the social worker. During his hospitalization, Joe experienced auditory hallucinations, suicidal and homicidal thoughts, and major depression. Joe's insurance coverage was set to expire on July 12. As that date neared, Dr. Barnhill decided that a blood test was needed to determine the proper dosage of a drug that he was prescribing for Joe. The blood test was scheduled for July 13 so Dr. Barnhill requested that the hospital administrator allow Joe to stay at Charter Hospital until July 14. This was agreed provided Mr. and Mrs. Muse sign a promissory note to pay for the two extra days. However,

---

18 *Id.* at 311.

19 *Id.* at 311.

20 *Id.* at 312.

21 452 S.E.2d 589 (N.C. App. 1995).

the test results did not come back from the lab until July 15; nevertheless, Joe was discharged on July 14. He was referred to the Guilford County Area Mental Health, Mental Retardation and Substance Abuse Authority for outpatient treatment. On July 22, Joe began outpatient treatment at the Mental Health Authority where he was seen by Dr. Slonaker, a clinical psychologist. Two days later, Joe again met with Dr. Slonaker. He failed to show for his July 30 appointment, and the next day Joe took a fatal overdose of one of his prescribed drugs.

The evidence at trial included the testimony of Charter Hospital employees and outside experts. Nurse Garzon testified that Charter Hospital's policy is to discharge patients when their insurance expired. As he explained, when the issue of insurance came up in treatment team meetings, plans were made to discharge the patient. Nurse Garzon testified, they would state, "So and so is to be discharged. We must do this."[22] Nurse Garzon further testified that when he returned from vacation and noted that Joe was no longer at the hospital, he asked several employees why Joe had been discharged and they all responded that he was discharged because his insurance had expired.

Jane Sims, a former staff member at Charter Hospital, testified that several employees expressed alarm about Joe's impending discharge, but a therapist had explained that Joe could no longer stay at the hospital because his insurance had expired. Ms. Sims also testified that Dr. Barnhill had misgivings about discharging Joe, which were apparent to everyone.

One of plaintiffs' experts testified that based on a study regarding the length of patient stays at Charter Hospital, in his opinion patients were discharged based on insurance, regardless of their medical condition. Other experts testified that in light of Joe's serious condition when he was discharged, the expiration of insurance coverage must have caused Dr. Barnhill to discharge Joe. The experts concluded that Charter Hospital's policies and practices were below the standard of care and caused Joe's death. They required physicians to discharge patients when their insurance benefits expired and that interfered with the exercise of Dr. Barnhill's medical judgment.

The parents also sought punitive damages because Charter Hospital engaged in conduct that was willful or wanton. In North Carolina, an act is willful "when it is done purposely and deliberately in violation of the law, or when it is done knowingly and of set purpose, or when the mere will has free play, without yielding to reason."[23] Conduct is considered wanton when it is done "of wicked purpose, or when it is done needlessly, with reckless indifference to the rights of others."[24] The court concluded "that the jury could have reasonably

22 *Id.* at 475.

23 *Id.* at 475.

24 *Id.*

found from the above-stated evidence that Charter Hospital acted knowingly and of set purpose and with reckless indifference to the rights of others."[25]

The jury found that Charter Hospital was negligent for having a policy or practice that required physicians to discharge patients when their insurance expired, and that this policy interfered with the exercise of the medical judgment of Dr. Barnhill. It awarded plaintiffs compensatory damages of approximately $1,000,000 and punitive damages of $2,000,000 against Charter Hospital. No damages were awarded against Dr. Barnhill. Although the jury also awarded punitive damages of $4,000,000 against Charter Medical Corporation, the appellate court reversed that award.

What is a hospital's duty to an involuntarily committed patient? This was the issue addressed by the court in *Marvel v. County of Erie.*[26] Upon arriving at the Emergency Department of Erie County Medical Center (ECMC), Amos Marvel was assessed by a nurse who placed him in wrist restraints until he could be seen by a physician. The nurse applied the restraints without a physician's order because Mr. Marvel was involuntarily committed, appeared intoxicated, and was threatening to leave. The nurse was aware of ECMC's policy requiring that patients in restraints and must be kept under constant supervision. Nor, did the nurse summon a physician, which was also contrary to ECMC's Policy. The Policy further required that a patient's restraints should be checked every 30 minutes and that an assessment of the patient's condition be made at least every 15 minutes and documented. Mr. Marvel's medical record did not reflect that such procedures were followed.

Mr. Marvel was eventually seen by a resident who failed to check Mr. Marvel's restraints during the 5–10 minutes that he was with him. Approximately 5–15 minutes after the resident left, Mr. Marvel, freed himself from his restraints, ran through the hospital, hung off the balcony, and fell more than 20 feet to the ground below.

Mr. Marvel contends that he was not provided with the "constant supervision" as required under State law and ECMC's policy. Because the term "constant supervision" was not defined in either the law or the policy, there were different interpretations of it provided at trial. The court concluded that the jury had sufficient evidence to find that ECMC failed to provide constant supervision in light of the information available that Mr. Marvel was suffering from depression, was under psychiatric treatment, had been drinking, and was violent and uncontrollable. The evidence was sufficient that Mr. Marvel was not provided with the requisite supervision and that he was left alone long enough to enable him to free himself from his restraints and run through the hospital.

25 *Id.*

26 762 N.Y.S.2d 753 (N.Y. A.D. 2003).

SECTION 9-4: HOME HEALTH

The medical conditions of patients now treated in their homes have markedly changed. Treatments that were experimental in hospitals a few years ago are now routinely performed in homes. Patients are discharged from hospitals in much more acute states, requiring high tech procedures and more intense follow-up care.

The same legal principles and concerns of nurses in other settings are applicable to home health nurses. However, there is a greater responsibility placed upon these nurses by virtue of them being more independent and autonomous than nurses in other settings. For example, appropriately monitoring a patient's condition and timely notifying a physician of significant changes is even more critical in home health care because the physician will not independently be assessing the patient.

Having appropriately qualified staff has become quite critical in home health care in light of the complex patients and treatments required by these patients. As a result, hiring appropriate staff and maintaining their competency must be a high priority. Verification of education and credentials must be clearly documented. References need to be contacted and these contacts documented. At least annually there should be an evaluation of the employee's competency, including verification of the employee's ability to perform technical skills. Ongoing education must be made available to maintain competency and to provide the necessary information regarding new equipment or procedures.

Home health agencies must have clearly defined admission policies for determining what patients they will accept. Any limitations on patients or treatments that the agency will provide must be clearly stated to avoid accepting a patient for whom the appropriate standard of care cannot be provided. When the agency accepts the referral of a patient, the duty is then established to provide the appropriate standard of care. If it cannot be determined whether a patient meets the admission policy without assessing the patient or obtaining further information, the patient should not be accepted as a referral until verification of appropriateness can be made.

A factor that must be included in the admission policy is determining what staff are required to provide services to that patient. The issues are whether the agency has appropriately qualified staff, and whether they are available to render the care and treatment to the patient within the required time period.

When equipment is needed for a patient, the agency must ascertain that staff know how to use the equipment. Additionally, if the agency is responsible for providing equipment, there must be verification of its availability. Where the agency utilizes another company to provide equipment, it must be clearly delineated as to who has responsibility for what aspect of the equipment.

Included in the admission policy must be clearly delineated discharge criteria for determining when a patient is to be discharged from the agency. Appropriate reasons for discharging a patient from an agency include the failure to have required physician monitoring, the failure to meet legal requirements for reimbursement, the failure to comply with or accept treatment, the failure to pay for the agency's services, the need for services the agency cannot provide, actual or threatened violence against home health care providers, mutual agreement that the patient be discharged, or the patient no longer needs the services of the agency. In addition to defined discharge criteria, the agency has the right to terminate a relationship with a patient for any reason when it is deemed to be in the best interest of either the agency or the patient.

What becomes critical is how the relationship is terminated. The failure to properly terminate a relationship could result in allegations of abandonment and malpractice. The patient must be given notice of the intent to terminate the relationship with a reasonable period of time to obtain any services that may be needed from another agency or provider. There is no clearly defined "reasonable time period;" rather, it depends upon the reason for terminating the relationship and the patient's condition. After advising the patient of the intent to terminate the relationship, prior to the date of termination the agency must continue to provide services to the patient as needed. If the patient needs to obtain services from someone else, it is appropriate for the agency to provide several suggestions where the patient can obtain those services. It is not recommended that an agency provide the patient with only one referral. In the event that the patient accepts that suggested referral and ultimately receives care that is below the standard, it is possible that the agency has liability based on the referral of the patient to that provider or agency.

In the notice of termination, advise the patient of the reason for terminating the relationship. The notice of termination must be in writing. While it is typically recommended that such notice be sent by certified mail, return receipt requested, in the event that the patient is unable to pick up mail at the post office, that may not be a practical method of delivery. Alternative methods would include hand-delivering the notice and having the patient sign a written acknowledgment of receipt of the notice, or have the notice delivered to the patient's home through a mail or delivery service.

Have written policies regarding termination that address what factors will justify terminating patient relationships, how much notice must be given, all parties to whom notice will and may be provided, and how notice is to be communicated.

The right of home health nurses to terminate a patient was the issue addressed in *Couch v. Visiting Home Care Service.*[27] John Couch was diagnosed

---

27 746 A.2d 1029 (N.J. App. 2000).

with MS for which he had been receiving skilled intermittent nursing services. Since 1998, Mr. Couch had received twice daily two hour visits from a certified home health aid, and visits of a shorter duration by a registered nurse once or twice daily, totaling about 33 hours each week. Mr. Couch became quadriplegic and developed a severe pressure sore on his buttocks. Surgery was performed and the surgeon encouraged Mr. Couch to obtain in-patient care. However, Mr. Couch resisted, explaining that remaining in his home was his "form of being independent."

Subsequently VHCS determined that Mr. Couch required care beyond their capabilities and notified him that "we will no longer be able to provide . . . services to you after March 24, due to the unsafe home care situation and your increasing need for more assistance than our home health aides can legally provide." Mr. Couch then sued VHCS, seeking to enjoin it from terminating his in-home skilled nursing and home health aid services.

At trial, the court noted that health care providers are free to refuse to participate and to withdraw from a case when the patient selects a course of treatment that the health care providers feel is inappropriate or unsafe. The court also recognized that Mr. Couch was competent and capable of deciding whether to enter a nursing home. The court concluded that if in the professional judgment of the home health nurses they cannot properly and ethically continue their care, they were entitled to terminate their treatment of Mr. Couch after providing him with a reasonable time in which to make alternative arrangements.

SECTION 9-5: LONG TERM CARE

In 1987, Congress enacted the Nursing Home Quality Reform Act which made comprehensive and fundamental changes in the way long-term care facilities deliver services, staff their facilities, are inspected by government agencies, and are sanctioned when their services do not meet standards set forth in the Act. This legislation substantially upgraded the quality of patient care in long-term care facilities and provides the blueprint for the future of long-term care. Under this Act, long-term care facilities must now comply with more than one hundred requirements.

A significant aspect of the Act was to strengthen the protection of the rights of residents and to expand those rights. These include the right to privacy, the right to receive notice before a change in room or roommate, the right to meet with other patients in organized groups, the right to voice grievances about care, the right to choose a personal attending physician, the right to participate in planning personal care and treatment, and the right to be free from physical and mental abuse, corporal punishment, involuntary seclusion, and physical and chemical restraints imposed for purposes of discipline or convenience. Another requirement is that psychopharmacologic drugs may be ordered by a physician only as part of a plan designed to eliminate or modify the symptoms for which the drugs are prescribed. An independent external consultant must, at least annually, review the appropriateness of the drug plan for each resident for whom these drugs are prescribed.

In July 1995, a new resident right became effective. This requires that prior to or upon admission of a resident, the resident or the resident's legal representative must be informed about the right of the resident to accept or refuse medical or surgical treatment and to formulate an advance directive.

Any deviation from the requirements imposed by the Act or its implementing regulations is a deficiency. Depending on the scope and severity of the violation, deficiencies are subject to a wide array of remedies, ranging from a plan of correction to $10,000 per day civil fines. As a result, various committees within Centers for Medicare and Medicaid Services (CMS) as well as independent groups are overseeing implementation of the regulations.

If a long-term care facility fails to meet the federal standards, the government may also deny Medicaid and Medicare payments. Payments must be withheld if the facility is found to be substandard in three consecutive annual surveys. Where a facility is out of compliance with requirements and its deficiencies immediately jeopardize the health or safety of its residents, the state in which the facility is located must take immediate actions to remove the jeopardy and correct deficiencies by appointing a temporary management team for the facility.

One of the concerns with the regulations is that they are intended to identify care that will be characterized by surveyors as "substandard." According to the regulations, this determination will be based on an in-depth evaluation of care by specially trained surveyors who use a protocol that CMS has designed, tested, and validated. If a surveyor determines that a long-term care facility delivered deficient or substandard care, this will imply that the patient did not receive care entitled to him. It is likely that these surveys may be used as the basis for malpractice actions arising out of these occurrences. In criminal and civil cases, survey deficiency reports will be admitted as evidence of poor care.

The failure to monitor a resident who had a history of seizures was the issue for the court in *Hammack v. Lutheran Social Services of Michigan*[28]. Jerry Hammack was a thirty-year-old mildly retarded, seizure-prone developmentally disabled man living in the Tracey Augustana Home. The home is a semi-independent living situation for developmentally disabled individuals such as Mr. Hammack. Mr. Hammack's individual plan of service was developed with the goal of increasing his independence. Accordingly, Mr. Hammack could be left

---

28 535 N.W.2d 215 (Mich. App. 1995).

alone and unsupervised for up to five hours a day. The Nursing Health Care Plan contained directions for intervention and care of Mr. Hammack during his seizures. The Nursing Health Care Plan also provided that Mr. Hammack was not to be left alone while bathing because of his past seizure activity.

Mr. Hammack died while bathing. It was alleged that he had a seizure while in the tub and that his death could have been prevented if Veronica Keenan, an employee of the home, had monitored Mr. Hammack while he bathed. The lawsuit was brought against Ms. Keenan and the home for their negligence in appropriately monitoring Mr. Hammack. At trial, the defendants argued that they owed no duty to monitor Mr. Hammack while bathing. Yet defendants conceded that Mr. Hammack entrusted himself to their control and protection. The risk of harm to Mr. Hammack was anticipated as evident by the provision in the Nursing Health Care Plan that Mr. Hammack was not to bathe unsupervised. The danger of him using the bathtub was foreseeable, requiring the defendants to take reasonable precautions.[29] The court thus upheld the jury verdict awarding the estate of Mr. Hammack $1,000,000 based on the negligence of the defendants.

More frequently we are seeing plaintiffs seeking punitive damages in malpractice actions brought against long-term care facilities and providers. Punitive damages were awarded by the jury in *Convalescent Services, Inc. v. Schultz*.[30] This was an action brought against a nursing home based on its failure to properly monitor and treat the resident's decubitus ulcers.

Jacob Schultz was admitted to Bayou Glen Nursing Home on July 5, 1991. At that time, Mr. Schultz was 77 years old and suffered from end-stage Alzheimer's dementia. He was bedridden, incontinent, and his limbs were contracted.

On admission, Bayou Glen's nursing staff noted that Mr. Schultz had a large, very dark red area on his coccyx and buttock, classified as a Stage I or II decubitus ulcer. The ulcer worsened to at least Stage III when the skin surface broke open eleven days later, on July 16th. On August 25th, Mr. Schultz was hospitalized for aggressive treatment of the steadily deteriorating decubitus ulcer, which had increased in size and progressed to Stage IV, exposing the bone. Mr. Schultz underwent several surgical procedures, including debridement of dead tissue and placement of a surgical skin flap to cover the exposed bone. After being hospitalized for over three months, prolonged by infections after surgery, Mr. Schultz was released and admitted to another nursing facility.

The plaintiffs alleged that the nursing care at Bayou Glen was so substandard that it precipitated the deterioration of the decubitus ulcer, and that this

---

29 *Id.* at 218.

30 921 S.W.2d 731 (Tex. App. 1996).

deterioration and the resulting surgical intervention were preventable if proper care had been given. They alleged that Bayou Glen was negligent and grossly negligent.

In Texas, to establish gross negligence for the purpose of imposing punitive damages, there must be evidence that (1) the act or omission, viewed objectively from the standpoint of the actor, involved an extreme degree of risk, considering the probability and magnitude of the potential harm to others; and (2) the actor had actual, subjective awareness of the risk involved, but nevertheless proceeded in conscious indifference to the rights, safety, or welfare of others.[31] The "extreme degree of risk" is not satisfied by a remote possibility of injury or even a high probability of minor harm; rather, it requires the likelihood of serious injury to the resident.[32]

Plaintiff's expert witness, Dr. Taffet, testified that without proper treatment, the probability of a decubitus ulcer getting worse is very high, but with timely intervention there is a 95% probability of preventing the ulcer from worsening. Dr. Taffet expressed his opinion that the nursing staff at Bayou Glen created an extreme risk to Mr. Schultz through its lack of care. One of the major complaints was that the medical records did not show that the nursing staff had turned Mr. Schultz every two hours. According to Dr. Taffet, if a patient with a Stage I ulcer is not turned every two hours, the ulcer will become a Stage III or Stage IV.

Nurse Theeck, Bayou Glen's Director of Nursing, testified that to prevent a decubitus ulcer from becoming worse, the nurses should follow a protocol of bathing, turning and repositioning, using a Spenco mattress, and ensuring that the nutritional needs of the resident are met. As Nurse Theeck recognized, when Mr. Schultz was admitted with a large red area on his buttock and coccyx, "bells and whistles" should go off for a nurse treating Mr. Schultz. She agreed that this red area was the beginning of what could be a serious problem if timely intervention was not initiated. Nurse Theeck acknowledged that it is incumbent on the nursing staff to take measures to prevent decubitus ulcers from becoming worse, and without proper treatment, the ulcers will worsen most of the time. She also admitted that the nursing staff were familiar with the treatment necessary for those with Alzheimer's disease, those who were incontinent, and those who were bedridden. As this testimony reflects, Bayou Glen had actual, subjective awareness of the risk to Mr. Schultz.

Nurse Theeck acknowledged that the medical records are the best evidence of the care that was given. From a review of Mr. Schultz's medical record, there is evidence that Bayou Glen's conduct, in this case its omissions, led to deterio-

---

31 *Id.* at 735.

32 *Id.*

ration of the decubitus ulcer and the probability of serious injury to Mr. Schultz because of Bayou Glen's failure to:

1. Turn Mr. Schultz every two hours to prevent the decubitus ulcer from developing into a life-threatening condition;
2. Notify Mr. Schultz' physician, Dr. Wall, about the decubitus ulcer until July 16th when it had progressed to Stage III;
3. Follow physician's orders by providing daily whirlpool baths on July 16, 17, 23, 24, 25, and 27;
4. Ensure that Mr. Schultz received sufficient nutrition to permit healing;
5. Provide a Spenco mattress to relieve pressure on the decubitus ulcer; and
6. Timely document Mr. Schultz' progress on a skin assessment flow chart.

The court concluded that it was reasonable to infer from the failure to document these items of care that they were not provided. "Contrary to Bayou Glen's argument, we do not find it equally likely that the nurses provided the necessary care but failed to note it on Schultz's chart."[33] That care was not given was also supported by the rapid deterioration of Mr. Schultz over an eleven day period. Although Bayou Glen argued that Mr. Schultz's condition deteriorated even with proper care being provided, the evidence offered was so weak as to do no more than create a "mere suspicion of its existence." This "legally constitutes no evidence."[34] "To conclude otherwise would encourage lack of documentation in medical records to avoid a finding of failure to give proper care."[35]

Nurse Theeck acknowledged that Bayou Glen's Policy required nurses to make notes of observations of patients during each of the three shifts for twenty-four hour period. However, there are no nursing notes for Mr. Schultz for July 9, 10, 11, 13, 14, or 15. There is also evidence that Bayou Glen may have falsified records. On a State-required reporting sheet dated July 16th, Bayou Glen indicated Mr. Schultz had no decubitus ulcers when by that date Mr. Schultz's ulcer had progressed to Stage III. Its records also show that lunch and dinner were provided to Mr. Schultz on August 25, even though he was discharged from Bayou Glen at 9:15 that morning. Bayou Glen also attempted to cover up the fact that it failed to provide sufficient nourishment to Mr. Schultz by changing its records to show that he was only 5'4" instead of 5'10" or 5'11" as other records and trial testimony showed.

---

33 *Id.* at 736.
34 *Id.*
35 *Id.*

Ms. Burdine, a State inspector who investigated the complaint made by Mr. Schultz's family, testified that violations of the Nurse Practice Act showed a conscious disregard by the nurses for the health and welfare of residents. There was evidence to establish that Bayou Glen nurses were guilty of the following acts of unprofessional conduct cited in the Nurse Practice Act:

1. Failing to institute nursing intervention to stabilize a patient's condition or prevent complications;
2. Knowingly or consistently failing to accurately report or document a resident's symptoms, responses, progress, medications, or treatment;
3. Knowingly or consistently failing to make entries or make false entries in records pertaining to the giving of medications, treatments, or nursing care; and
4. Failing to administer medications or treatments in a responsible manner.

Mr. Schultz's son testified that although he visited his father frequently, no one at Bayou Glen informed him or any other family members of the existence of his father's decubitus ulcer. It was not until the ulcer had progressed to Stage IV that the son discovered its presence when he noticed a foul odor. This failure to keep the family informed was also in violation of Bayou Glen's Policy and additional evidence to support Bayou Glen's conscious indifference for its residents.

The court concluded that Bayou Glen's knowing violation of its own Policies, the failure of its nurses to comply with the Nurse Practice Act, the apparent falsification of records, and the disregard for physician's orders constituted evidence of "conscious disregard for the risk of serious harm to Mr. Schultz." As the court noted:

> Schultz was totally dependent on Bayou Glen for all activities of daily life. He was helpless to even complain about any severe pain he was suffering. This vulnerability enhances the seriousness of the risks to which Bayou Glen's conduct exposed Schultz. Bayou Glen was responsible for caring for Schultz's needs and protecting him from injury. Through its omissions, Bayou Glen permitted his condition to deteriorate and develop into a life-threatening situation. It consistently violated its own policies and nursing procedures. Bayou Glen permitted Schultz to rapidly deteriorate without even informing his family of the existence of a decubitus ulcer and the seriousness of the risk it posed. These actions certainly offend a public sense of justice and propriety warranting the imposition of damages both as punishment and as a deterrent to such practices in an effort to ensure quality care for elderly persons in nursing homes.[36]

---

36 *Id.* at 740.

The court thus upheld the jury's verdict against Bayou Glen, assessing $380,000 in actual damages and $850,000 in punitive damages.

A jury also decided punitive damages were warranted in a malpractice and wrongful death lawsuit brought against two physicians and their medical group.[37] On February 7, 1991, Edna Danner, age 85, was admitted to the Parkway Care Home under the medical care of the Blue Valley Medical Group. She entered the home able to walk with a walker and carry on a normal conversation. She had undergone recent back surgery and was diabetic; however, her family fully expected that she would recuperate and return home.

Seven months later, Mrs. Danner was transferred to a hospital dehydrated, disoriented, malnourished, and suffering from decubitus ulcers. She was treated in the hospital for two weeks and returned to the nursing home. By November 1991, Mrs. Danner was in a vegetative state and had advanced decubitus ulcers on her heels and backside. She subsequently died on February 10, 1992.

The allegations were that Blue Valley and Dr. Murray had fraudulently represented to Mrs. Danner that Mr. Gladstone Tucker was a licensed physician when in fact he was not. Mr. Tucker received an M.D. degree in the Soviet Union, but failed U.S. medical board exams four times. However, the Blue Valley Medical Group billed Mr. Tucker's services under the name of Dr. Murray. This obviously violated Federal laws by billing Medicare for Mr. Tucker's services.

There was also evidence that while treating Mrs. Danner, Mr. Tucker and Dr. Murray were serving about thirty-four nursing homes and managing care for over 1,100 patients per month. Testimony reflected that Dr. Murray saw up to eighty-five patients a day.

There was additional evidence that Mr. Tucker and Dr. Murray ordered unnecessary lab tests for Mrs. Danner. Of particular interest, these tests were performed by Johnson County Medical Lab, whose president was Dr. Robert LaHue, also the president of Blue Valley Medical Group.

The jury returned a verdict of $635,000 against the defendants. They also recommended punitive damages. Pursuant to Kansas law, punitive damages must be set by the judge in a separate hearing. The Wyandotte County District Court Judge set punitive damages at $300,000 against Blue Valley Medical Group and $40,000 against Dr. Murray. In his order, Judge Sieve stated:

> The jury found that Edna Danner endured pain and suffering and ultimately death due to the negligent treatment afforded her by the defendants. At least part of that negligence arose out of defendants allowing her to be treated by an unlicensed physician who had failed his licens-

---

37 *A Jury Awards $635,000 plus Punitives Against Blue Valley Medical Group*, 12 KINH News 1 (May–June 1994).

ing test four times. All of this was within the knowledge of the defendants. One can hardly minimize the effect that defendants' fraud had upon the health and life of Mrs. Danner. In light of this tragic result, the jury chose to punish the wrongdoers and send a message intended to deter others who might be inclined to conduct themselves in the manner of these defendants.[38]

Issues may arise as to the appropriateness of a resident to be admitted into or to be discharged from a long term care facility. Under both Section 504 of the Rehabilitation Act of 1973 and the Americans with Disabilities Act, no otherwise qualified individual shall, solely by reason of her or his disability, be excluded from the participation in, be denied the benefits of, or be subjected to discrimination in any program or activity.

Whether the plaintiff was discriminated against and denied admission was the issue for the court in *Grubbs v. Medical Facilities of America, Inc.*[39] The plaintiff, Judith Grubbs, was 48 years old and weighed 359 lb. She had multiple sclerosis and numerous other medical conditions. She had lost sight in one eye and was essentially immobile. As a result of her condition, Ms. Grubbs required specialized care, termed "subacute" care. Ms. Grubbs was denied admission at two nursing homes operated by Medical Facilities of America because of her weight and medical condition. Neither of the nursing homes were equipped nor licensed to provide subacute care.

The issue for the court was whether Ms. Grubbs was an "otherwise qualified" individual able to meet all the program's requirements in spite of her handicap. The court concluded that Ms. Grubbs was not "otherwise qualified" for admission to either of the nursing homes since they did not offer subacute care. By her own admission, this is the type of care she required, and she had been determined eligible for Medicaid subacute care payments. Although there is an obligation for a facility to make a reasonable accommodation for a person with a disability, "an accommodation is not reasonable when it imposes an undue financial hardship . . . or requires a fundamental alteration in the nature of the program."[40] For the nursing homes to have admitted Ms. Grubbs, they would have to become subacute care providers. Such an accommodation is clearly not required under the Rehabilitation Act or the Americans with Disabilities Act.[41]

Once a resident is admitted to a facility, the facility may not discharge the resident involuntarily without complying with State and Federal discharge criteria.

38 *A Judge Sets Punitive Damages at $340,000*, 13 KINH News 4 (Winter 1995).

39 879 F. Supp. 588 (W.D. Va. 1995).

40 *Id.* at 590.

41 *Id.* at 591.

SECTION 9-6: MATERNAL-CHILD

A multimillion dollar verdict was rendered in favor of a severely brain-damaged 20-month old child by a Los Angeles jury that was greatly influenced by a nurse's statement that she was "too busy to auscultate the fetal heart rate" during twenty-two minutes in the delivery room.[42] The patient's mother was at term when she was brought to the defendant hospital, Centenela Hospital Medical Center of Los Angeles, at 6:00 a.m. Her membranes spontaneously ruptured at 9:00 a.m. and there was slight meconium. Because of slow progress, the patient's obstetrician started her on Pitocin at noon. She was on an electronic fetal heart monitor, which was routine at the hospital.

About 3:30 p.m. some subtle variable decelerations developed. At 5:45 p.m., there was a dramatic late deceleration down to a heart rate of 60 which lasted for six minutes before the heart rate recovered to the baseline. The cervix was fully dilated at 6:00 p.m. The mother was told to push and with every contraction over the next two hours the monitor showed severe variable decelerations. At 8:00 p.m. the mother was taken to the delivery room. The electronic fetal heart monitor was disconnected and was not reapplied in the delivery room because there was none available. Thus, over the next twenty-two minutes until the baby was delivered, the fetal heart tones were not auscultated.

On delivery at 8:22 p.m., the Apgar scores were 0 at one minute, 3 at five minutes, and 7 at ten minutes. Seizures developed soon after birth and the initial EEG was flat. It was recommended that the baby be taken off of life support but the family refused. The patient improved and was discharged after nineteen days. She now has a gastrostomy feeding tube, severe mental retardation, and spastic quadriplegia.

Shortly before trial, the obstetrician settled for $956,000. Thus, at trial, the Medical Center was the only defendant.

There was testimony concerning the training obstetrical nurses receive in interpreting electronic fetal heart monitors. There was expert testimony from a nurse and obstetrician asserting that, in view of the obvious and continuing abnormality on the fetal heart monitor strip, the nurse should have intervened and obtained help. It was clear that the nurse had an independent duty to protect the interests of the mother and fetus.

With regard to the twenty-two minutes in the delivery room, the obstetrical nurse who was with the mother at this time conceded that a protocol required her to auscultate the fetal heart rate every five minutes. She testified that she was just too busy to do it even once. Of significance, the one area of testimony where the jury asked for the court reporter's notes to be read to them after they

---

42 Los Angeles County Superior Court, No. YC012998, 24 *Professional Liability Newsletter* (February 1994).

began their deliberations concerned the nurse's admission that she should have been monitoring the fetal heart rate in the delivery room. Trial observers felt this may have been the most important evidence from the jury's standpoint. The plaintiff's expert witness emphasized that the zero Apgar score at one minute indicated a rapid deterioration of the baby during this critical time when no fetal heart rate was determined.

Because the bulk of the jury's award was an annuity, the precise value of the verdict was unclear but may have been as much as $10,000,000. However, the case was resolved with payment of an undisclosed amount, thought to be approximately $3,000,000.

A medical malpractice action was brought against a Hospital for its alleged negligence that resulted in the death of a newborn.[43] The allegations were that the Hospital was aware that the unborn child had passed meconium *in utero*; that the Hospital knew or should have known that delivery was imminent; that the Hospital should have moved Mrs. Murdock to the delivery room; that the Hospital should have made available all necessary devices and instruments to suction the nasopharynx of the baby before his shoulders were delivered; and that a pediatrician adept and trained in resuscitation should have been present at delivery.

Kathy Murdock entered Wetly Hospital, ready to give birth. She was placed in a labor room and examined by Dr. Wilson. Dr. Wilson was aware that Mrs. Murdock had previously given birth to a baby with severe congenital birth defects and that tests had indicated similar problems with this pregnancy. At 2:00 a.m., Mrs. Murdock was instructed by Nurse Slicer to call when she had an urge to push. At 2:27 a.m., Mrs. Murdock had a need to push and the cervix was at nine centimeters. At 3:00 a.m., a sterile vaginal exam was performed and the notes indicate that the cervix was complete. Mrs. Murdock was instructed to start pushing. At 3:05 a.m., Mrs. Murdock continued to push and stated that she could not stop pushing. At 3:05 a.m. the baby was delivered. As predicted, Jesse was born with severe congenital birth defects. He also had meconium in his mouth. However, Jesse was not suctioned immediately after birth. Nurse Slicer and Nurse Turner could not remember whether a suctioning device was available in the labor room.

Jesse was immediately taken to the nursery. Nurse Burroughs testified that when she received Jesse, she put a bag and mask over his face and started forcing air down his throat. This evidently forced the meconium down farther into the lungs. Jesse was subsequently suctioned in the nursery, approximately eight to ten minutes after birth. The evidence was that prior to this, he was not getting oxygen, which resulted in brain damage, and ultimately his death.

---

43 *Texarkana Memorial Hospital, Inc. v. Murdock*, 903 S.W.2d 868 (Tex. App. 1995).

At trial, Nurse Roberts testified that she was familiar with the standard of care expected of labor and delivery nurses, and she believed that the nurses did not timely take Mrs. Murdock to the delivery room. She also testified that the nurses did not have the necessary equipment available when Jesse was delivered. There was evidence that when Mrs. Murdock's membranes ruptured at 11:03 p.m., the fluid was stained with meconium. This was more than four hours before the delivery and gave the nurses notice to prepare to avoid meconium aspiration at the time of the delivery. Nurse Roberts testified that a registered nurse would have known that meconium is a risk factor because if it is inhaled or aspirated, it will cause problems. Therefore, the infant must be suctioned at the time of delivery.

Both Nurse Slicer and Nurse Turner testified that their general procedure was to notify the physician when the patient has an urge to push and a vaginal exam shows the patient to be complete. However, there was no documentation in Mrs. Murdock's medical record that Dr. Wilson was ever notified.

Dr. Caldwell testified that the nurses failed to adhere to the standard of care required of the situation by allowing a multiparous patient to push in the labor room, by failing to timely notify the attending obstetrician, and by failing to provide the necessary equipment when they knew that there was meconium-stained fluid.

Mrs. Murdock was awarded $500,000 by the jury because of the hospital's negligence.

The failure to screen a newborn for PKU resulted in damages totalling $5.5 million.[44] Brian McKee was born on May 1, 1977, at Humana Hospital. On that date, Kentucky law required hospitals to perform a PKU test on each newborn infant no sooner than twenty-four hours after birth. The test requires blood to be drawn from the infant's heel and placed directly on filter paper that is provided by and returned to the State laboratory for testing. The blood specimen is analyzed and the results then are returned to the hospital. The blood of an infant who suffers from PKU will show an elevated level of phenylalanine, which is an amino acid formed from protein. PKU is a metabolic disorder that causes the body to be unable to process phenylalanine and the ingestion of protein causes abnormal levels of phenylalanine to accumulate in the child's body. This damages the developing central nervous system, especially the brain, resulting in mental retardation and a likelihood of major seizures. The harmful accumulation of phenylalanine can easily be prevented if a diagnosis of PKU is made at or near birth, as treatment is simply restricting the child's dietary intake of

---

44 *Humana of Kentucky, Inc. v. McKee*, 834 S.W.2d 711 (Ky. App. 1992). This is an example of the extended statute of limitations for an injury sustained by a minor.

proteins. With timely treatment, a child with PKU can be expected to lead a normal, healthy, and productive life.

Brian's medical record indicates that on May 19, 1977, when he was eighteen days old, Hospital personnel noted in his record that the State laboratory reported that Brian's PKU test result was negative. Although developmental problems were subsequently noted during Brian's infancy and early childhood, his parents and physicians assumed that he was progressing slowly or that he was suffering from some vague psychological difficulties. Subsequently, it became apparent that Brian had suffered significant developmental delays. In 1983, he was diagnosed as having PKU.

The evidence was that there was no entry in Brian's medical record by either a nurse or a laboratory technician to show that a blood specimen was ever taken from Brian. His medical record reflected only that upon Brian's birth, the doctor ordered that a PKU test be performed on the day of discharge and a notation following that order indicated that the McKees were charged for the test when the order was transmitted from the nursery to Hospital's laboratory. The record also shows that the night nursery staff forwarded the test order to the laboratory, and that the nurse made an entry in the nursery log book indicating that a PKU test would be performed.

Sally New, Humana's Director of Nursing Administration, testified that the fact of taking a blood specimen for a PKU test was a significant piece of clinical information. She affirmed the existence of standards require that entries of all significant pieces of clinical information were made in patient medical records.

The McKees introduced evidence of the Hospital's written "PKU Procedures" that provides a step-by-step outline of the actions Hospital personnel are required to take in obtaining PKU samples. Brian's medical record reflects that these procedures were not met as follows:

1. The spaces for a date and time on the requisition slip were left blank, as well the space for the initials of the person who drew the blood, and the laboratory technician did not stamp the requisition slip with the laboratory timer clock;

2. The laboratory technician did not date or initial the State laboratory form for PKU screening; and

3. According to the records of Brian's physician, the latter received no letter from Humana regarding the test results.

The morning of the alleged test, May 4, 1977, was evidently an unusually busy one and apparently a laboratory technician drew blood from several infants for PKU testing and placed that blood on the filter paper portions of the lab

219

forms. This unidentified technician failed to record his or her initials on the requisition slips or the screening cards, or to stamp the slips in any of the seven cases. Moreover, although each lab form is supposed to be marked with the infant's name and patient number, in Brian's case the night nurse mistakenly entered on the form the patient number for Brian's mother rather than for Brian.

After obtaining the blood specimen for the PKU test, the laboratory personnel were instructed to enter the child's name, patient number, and other data into a PKU log book. The log book entry for Brian erroneously included his mother's patient number rather than Brian's.

Dr. Strand, Humana's Director of Pathology, testified that hospital procedures require the laboratory technician to obtain the lab forms from the nursery staff, and to then locate and identify the babies whose blood will be drawn. Each baby's bassinet contains the baby's patient number, which the technician matches to the baby's patient number as shown on the lab form. The technician does not rely upon either the baby's name or the patient number shown on the requisition slip. The evidence was that the unidentified technician who was attempting to find a baby boy with the erroneous patient number of Mrs. McKee would not have found Brian, as he was in a bassinet with his correct patient number. Bernice Brown, a laboratory employee, testified that she noticed when Brian's lab form was brought to the laboratory that it was marked with the wrong patient number. She called the nursery to point out this mistake, but apparently nothing more was done to follow up this call.

At trial, the McKees introduced into evidence guidelines of the Joint Commission on Accreditation of Hospitals and certain federal regulations. Both Dr. Strand and Dr. Mabry testified that essentially all of the JCAHO guidelines and Federal regulations set forth reasonable standards that a hospital should follow when complying with its duty of ordinary care in drawing blood specimens from patients. The court found that these were evidence of the procedures that a reasonably prudent hospital would follow in drawing a patient's blood specimen. It also gave the jury reasonable criteria to utilize in determining whether the procedures that the Hospital claimed it followed in Brian's case complied with its duty of ordinary care.

There is also an issue as to whether the notation that a negative PKU test was received on May 19, 1977, was actually *not* entered in Brian's Hospital record until after Dr. Mabry requested Brian's records some six years later. Beth Harp, an employee in the Kentucky Division of Maternal and Child Health, testified she received a telephone call from Hospital's Medical Records Director, Judy Owens. Ms. Harp testified that Ms. Owens asked whether a positive PKU test had ever been obtained on Brian. Ms. Owens reported that she had Brian's chart and there was nothing written about a PKU test—there was nothing in the chart, either a positive or a negative test result. Ms. Harp further testified that

Ms. Owens told her that normally the Hospital places a copy of the PKU test result in the chart. She also reported that the clinic where Brian's physician worked also had nothing in the chart.

Brian's specialist for his PKU treatment, Dr. Mabry, apparently received no answer to two routine requests for Brian's Hospital medical record after he began to treat Brian in 1983, and did not finally receive the medical record until after the litigation had been initiated. At that time, Brian's Hospital medical record contained a written notation that showed a negative PKU test result was received. Bernice Brown, the laboratory technician who earlier had attempted to look into the suspected mistake as to Brian's hospital number, conceded that she had no actual memory of receiving and transcribing a negative test result.

The court concluded that substantive evidence was established and supported at trial including the following facts and reasonable inferences in their favor:

1. There is not one record entry that a PKU blood specimen was taken from Brian, nor is there a record of the laboratory technician who would have taken it, nor the time taken.

2. The laboratory technician taking any blood specimens had only the lab form incorrectly listing Brian's Hospital number. Any laboratory technician looking for a baby in the nursery with the Hospital number for Mrs. McKee would not have found Brian.

3. The laboratory technician did not discover the error in the Hospital number, and must have *thought* he took a blood specimen from a baby with the Hospital number for Mrs. McKee on the specimen card titled Brian McKee. That blood specimen would not have been from Brian.

4. To assure the accuracy of the blood specimens, and to assure that they are taken from the correct patient, the Hospital's protocol required five steps which were not performed: no initials, time, or timer clock on the laboratory requisition slip, and no initials or date on the lab form.

5. When the specimen card bearing Brian's name, but not his blood, was delivered to the Hospital's pathology lab, the mistake in the source of the specimen was noted but never corrected.

6. In 1984, the Hospital's Director of Medical Records, well familiar with reading charts, advised an independent witness that Brian's Hospital chart did not indicate any result whatsoever of a PKU test.

7. The Hospital stonewalled Dr. Mabry when he twice requested Brian's birth record in 1983.

8. Mrs. McKee testified that she did not remember whether the band-aid she once saw on Brian's heel was from Brian's birth admission or his

admission two weeks later, when the chart indicated that Brian had a CBC test performed, which also would have required a heel stick and a band-aid.

9. The State laboratory had extensive quality control procedures assuring accurate administration of the PKU test. The State laboratory had extensive procedures to ensure the absence of testing error.

10. The Hospital admitted it knew of no evidence indicating neglect on the part of the State laboratory.

11. There is no basis for concluding that Brian might have been a "biologic variant," a 1 out of 300,000,000 chance.

The appellate court affirmed the jury's verdict finding Humana Hospital negligent and awarding Brian damages totaling $5.5 million.

When labor and delivery don't go as planned and the baby is compromised physically and/or mentally, is frequently legal actions are taken against the health care providers. Two factors most often cited in these claims are delay in the diagnosis of fetal distress and insufficient documentation. Since 1990, insurance company reported that 1 out of every 1,000 births involving an insured health care provider has lead to a malpractice claim or lawsuit.[45] Between 1987 and 1996, nurses were named in 70% of all claims that named non-physicians, and 14% of all claims.[46] In 1998, delay in diagnosing fetal distress was reported to be a factor in 88% of malpractice cases related to neurologically impaired newborns, up 41% from 10 years earlier.[47] What has been noticed is that the delay in diagnosing fetal distress is usually associated with insufficient documentation and lack of oral communication.

The Association of Women's Health, Obstetric and Neonatal Nurses (AWHONN) has identified standards for interpartum fetal heart monitoring as has the American College of Obstetricians and Gynecologists (ACOG). The standard strongly advises that all nurses who perform fetal assessment during the antepartum or intrapartum period complete a course of study that includes the physiologic interpretation of electronic fetal monitoring data and its implications for labor support.[48] The use and interpretation of electronic fetal monitoring often plays a crucial role in obstetrical malpractice claims.

---

45 Groff, H., *Understanding CRICO's Perinatal Claims*, 21 Forum 1 (2001).

46 Groff, H. and Martin, P., *CRICO's Claims Involving Non-Physician Employees*, 18 Forum 1 (1998).

47 Physician Insures Association of America, *Neurological Impairment in Newborns: A Malpractice Claims Study* (1998).

48 Association of Women's Health, Obstetric and Neonatal Nurses, *Fetal Assessment* (Position Statement) (2000).

The failure to detect fetal distress in a timely manner due to infrequency of the fetal monitoring tracing and failing to promptly inform the obstetrician of fetal distress are significant factors in claims alleging nursing negligence.[49]

An action was brought by the parents of a $4^1/_2$ year old female patient who suffered brain damage caused by Kernicterus, which results from an elevated bilirubin count, secondary to untreated jaundice.[50] Kernicterus is highly preventable if jaundice is timely and properly treated.

Krista was born at Newton Wellesley Hospital and was given a pediatric examination later that day. The following day the infant was discharged. When asked about the apparent jaundice, the nurse informed the mother that this was common, would increase the following day, and that she might want to call her pediatrician if the child became lethargic and stopped eating. On the following evening, Krista's bilirubin count escalated to the point where it resulted in Kernicterus. Krista sustained profound brain damage and suffers from cerebral palsy. The allegations against the nurse were failing to detain Krista for evaluation and testing, and failing to provide the parents with adequate discharge instructions. Evidence was that the nurse had her observation of the jaundice at the time of discharge. The medical testimony documented was undisputed that neonatal jaundice progresses from head to toe, and the standard method to assess the severity of the condition is to examine the infant's entire body. The defendant nurse conceded that it would be negligent to discharge Krista without first undressing her to determine how far down her body the jaundice had progressed; the nurse maintained that she had done such an evaluation. Krista's mother disputed this assertion, contended that the child was fully dressed and that only her face was visible when assessed by defendant nurse just prior to discharge. Krista's pediatrician was shown a photograph of Krista at the time of discharge which clearly depicted her obviously yellow pallor. The pediatrician testified that the defendant nurse should have notified her of the condition before allowing Krista to leave the hospital.

The severity of Krista's condition at the time a proper diagnosis was made strongly supported the parents' factual version of the events which occurred at the time of discharge. Krista's parents were very credible in their testimony as to what exactly occurred and what specifically was said at the time of discharge. The jury perceived them as being devoted and loving parents who would follow any and every instruction given them by the nurse on behalf of their child.

The evidence was undisputable that jaundice is easily detectable and easily reversible at any time up to the point where brain damage is sustained, under-

---

49 Connors, P.M., *High-Risk Perinatal Issues: Delay in the Diagnosis of Fetal Distress*, 9 Journal of Nursing Law 19 (2003).

50 *Lucas v. Loan*, RN, Case No.: MICV94-01888, (Middlesex County, Mass. May 1999).

scoring the particularly tragic nature of this case. The jury found for the plaintiffs and returned a verdict of $7,175,000: $4 million future medical cost; $1 million pain and suffering; $700,000 future lost wages; $600,000 emotional distress; and $75,000 to the parents for their loss of consortium. The plaintiffs also received prejudgment interest of $3, 325,000.

SECTION 9-7: OCCUPATIONAL HEALTH

With the expansion of the scope of practice of occupational health nurses, liability has increased. Occupational health nurses are heavily influenced by a multiplicity of Federal and State laws that govern occupational safety and health, worker's compensation, communicable disease reporting requirements, and the scope of practice of occupational health nurses through Nurse Practice Acts.

The law varies among the States as to whether independent actions for malpractice may be initiated against occupational health nurses. Some States allow such lawsuits while others take the position that the only recovery available to an injured employee is through worker's compensation. Other States allow the employee to elect to pursue a claim under worker's compensation or in a malpractice action.

A Federal law of importance to occupational health nurses is the Americans with Disabilities Act (ADA), which was enacted in 1990.[51] The goal of the Act is to end discrimination against persons with disabilities. The five sections of the Act are as follows:

Title I: *Employment*—The ADA prohibits entities from discriminating against a qualified individual with a disability in all aspects of employment.

Title II: *State and Local Government Services*—The ADA prohibits discrimination against individuals with disabilities in the provision of services, programs, and activities provided by state and local governments, including public transportation.

Title III: *Public Accommodations*—The ADA requires that private businesses must be accessible to persons with disabilities with varying requirements for existing facilities, alterations, and new construction.

Title IV: *Telecommunications*—The ADA requires that telecommunications relay services are available, to the extent possible, 24 hours a day for the deaf and hearing impaired.

Title V: *Miscellaneous Provisions*—These aspects of the ADA are generally applicable rules, employment specific applications, address required

---

51 42 U.S.C.S. § 12101 *et seq.*

accessibility to national wilderness areas, and applications to the Architectural and Transportation Barriers Compliance Board.

Title I is the most pertinent section of the ADA affecting occupational health nurses. They may become involved in determining whether an individual is qualified to perform the essential functions of the job with or without reasonable accommodation. The law requires that if a person has a disability, the employer is required to provide reasonable accommodations to enable the person to perform the job.

"Reasonable accommodation" is defined as modifications or adjustments:

1. To a job application or testing process that enable a qualified applicant with a disability to be considered for the position desired;
2. To the work environment or the manner or circumstances in which the job held or desired is customarily performed that enable an individual with a disability to perform the essential functions of the position; or
3. That enable an employee with a disability to enjoy equal benefits and privileges of employment as are enjoyed by similarly situated employees without disabilities.[52]

What is "reasonable" is determined on a case by case basis, depending upon factors such as the type and size of the business and what accommodation is necessary.

Another ADA provision requires that job applications and interviews, can't ask questions regarding the presence of any disabilities or the nature of any disability. Until a job offer has been made to an applicant, neither a medical nor a psychological examination may be performed. It is appropriate to extend an offer of employment *conditional* upon the results of the examinations. However, the examination must be required of all applications for that particular position.

Testing for illegal drugs is not prohibited since the use of illegal drugs is not protected under the ADA. The ADA also does not prohibit tests or examinations that are job related and consistent with business necessity.

Occupational health nurses are in a position to help the employer comply with the various aspects of the American with Disabilities Act. They are uniquely qualified to educate management and other employees regarding disabilities or medical conditions that may be erroneously perceived as constituting a disability.

Occupational health nurses are in positions where the employee's right to privacy and confidentiality becomes an issue with human resources or other department directors. An occupational health physician brought a wrongful

52 29 C.F.R. § 1630.2(o)(1).

discharge claim against her employer because of this issue.[53] The question presented is whether a physician whose employment is terminated because she refuses to share health information with individuals not authorized to have such information has a cause of action against her employer for wrongful discharge.

Dr. Horn alleges that on frequent occasions, various-named departments of the company directed her to provide them with confidential health information of employees "without those employees' consent or knowledge," and that the Vice President for Human Resources instructed her to "misinform employees regarding injuries or illnesses they were suffering were work related so as to curtail the number of workers compensation claims filed against the company." Dr. Horn refused to comply with these requests these and was shortly thereafter terminated from her employment. The Times alleged that Dr. Horn was terminated "due to economically induced restructuring of the department."

Dr. Horn testified that she was responsible for determining whether employee's injuries were work related and thus determining whether employees were eligible for workers compensation benefits. The Times argued that this was an evaluative and administrative corporate function; that Dr. Horn was performing "professional services in furtherance of their corporate responsibilities." The court disagreed with the Times, holding that "the determination of whether an injury is work-related is a diagnostic function and an integral part of the practice of medicine . . . which was at the very core of her employment."[54]

The Times further contended that confidentiality is not part of the professional code that is essential to the survival of the medical profession and that the physician-patient confidentiality obligation is not applicable here where "the employee-patient is fully aware that the physician is employed by the employer and thus has some duty to the employer as well."

There was evidence from the Council on Ethical and Judicial Affairs of the American Medical Association regarding industry-employed physicians. Such physicians are required to maintain patient confidentiality as physicians who are independent contractors. If an employee authorizes the release of health information to an employer or a potential employer, the physician should release only that information which is reasonably relevant to the employer's decision regarding that employee's ability to perform that work required by the job.[55]

In further noting that a physician's breach of patient confidentiality is grounds for suspension or revocation of license to practice medicine, the court upheld the right of Dr. Horn to pursue her wrongful discharge claim against The New York Times.

---

53 *Horn v. The New York Times*, 739 N.Y.S.2d 679 (N.Y.A.D.2002).

54 *Id.* at 683.

55 *Id.* at 685.

SECTION 9-8: SCHOOL HEALTH

The Individuals with Disabilities Education Act (IDEA) was created by Congress in response to the lack of educational opportunities for children with disabilities.[56] Within the past ten years, burdens on school districts to provide the educational opportunities, required by the IDEA have grown substantially and have frequently been the subject of court determinations. The majority of courts have held that school districts are not required to furnish full-time health related services to students with disabilities as the IDEA doesn't intend to impose such financial and administrative burdens upon States. Recently the United States Supreme Court ruled otherwise.

Garret is wheelchair bound and ventilator dependent. He therefore requires responsible individuals nearby to attend to certain physical needs during the school day. The School District declined to accept financial responsibility for the services Garret needs, believing that it was not legally obligated to provide continuous one-on-one nursing care. The significant issue in the case revolves around the analysis of "related services" and whether the services were excluded as "medical services."[57] The applicable Federal regulations require school districts to furnish "school health services" provided by a "qualified school nurse or other qualified person," but not "medical services," which are limited to services provided by a physician. As the Supreme Court previously held, "Services provided by a physician (other than for diagnostic and evaluation purposes) are subject to the medical services exclusion, but services that can be provided by a nurse or qualified lay person are not."[58] The Supreme Court had previously determined that the Secretary of Education had reasonably determined that determined that "medical services" refer to services that *must* be performed by a physician, and not to school health services.[59]

As the Supreme Court concluded, this case is about whether meaningful access to public schools will be assured as Congress intended. Since it is undisputed that the services at issue must be provided if Garret is to remain in school, the School District must fund such related services to guarantee that students like Garret are integrated into the public schools.

The refusal of a school health nurse to give a student a dosage of medication that exceeded the daily recommendation listed in the Physician's Desk Reference (PDR) resulted in a legal action against the school health nurse and

---

56 20 U.S.C. § 1400 *et seq.*

57 *Cedar Rapids Community School District v. Garret F.*, 119 S. Ct. 992 (1999).

58 *Id.* at 994.

59 *Id.* at 995. *See also, Irving Independent School District v. Tatro*, 468 U.S. 883, 1045. Ct. 337 (1984).

the School District.[60] Kelly has attention deficit hyperactivity disorder (ADHD) for which she is prescribed Ritalin. While the School District provides health services to students, including administration of prescription drugs during school hours, it has a written Policy against administering prescription drugs in an amount that exceeds the recommended daily dosage in the PDR. The recommended daily dosage for Ritalin for Kelly is 60mg. Kelly's physician had prescribed 100mg of Ritalin when Kelly arises in the morning and 40 mg at 3 pm. Thus, School Nurse Joyce Dreimeier, refused to give Kelly her afternoon dose.

When the School Board was approached by Kelly's parents, it offered several alteration, including alternation of Kelly's class schedule to permit early dismissal and home administration of both of Kelly's doses, or administration of Kelly's afternoon dose at school by one of her parents or someone designated by them. The parents were unhappy with the alternatives and brought an action alleging that the School District was violating the Rehabilitation Act and the American with Disabilities Act.

While recognizing the both the Rehabilitation Act and the ADA require the School District to "provide a free appropriate public education to each qualified handicapped person," the court concluded that it wasn't discriminatory to have objectively written policies limiting the administration of prescription medications only when the prescription exceeds the maximum dosage recommended in the PDR. There was certainly no evidence that the School District had disabilities in mind when formulating or implementing the Policies. While the DeBords argued that the School District's fears are invalid, the court defended the School District's position since it applies to all students regardless of disability. It is "a student's excess prescription, not the student's disability, that prevents the student from receiving medication from the school nurse."[61]

The court upheld the summary judgment granted in favor of the School District and the school health nurse based on the School District's Policy to refuse administrating excess doses of medication, which is rationally related to the legitimate State interest of protecting the health of students.

---

60 *DeBord v. Board of Education of the Ferguson/Florissant School District*, 126 F.3d 1102 (8th Cir. 1997).

61 *Id.* at 1105.

CHAPTER 10

Case Studies

SECTION 10-1: ELEMENTS OF LIABILITY

A. Mrs. Thomson

Mrs. Thomson is admitted to the hospital for treatment of a uterine fibroid tumor. Dr. Hardy removes it. Following surgery, Dr. Hardy administers an epidermal injection of sterile Durmorph for pain control. Mrs. Thomson is taken to the surgical floor, where you assume her care. Dr. Hardy orders monitoring by an RN every 30 minutes which you provide from 1:00 p.m. until 4:48 p.m. However the hospital has a "nursing service department labor and delivery policy" that provide guidelines for the use an apnea monitor for a patient treatment with an epidural injection of morphine.

- What is your *duty* to Mrs. Thompson?

- If you fail to notify Dr. Hardy of the policy requiring use of apnea monitor, have you committed *malpractice?*

- At 4:48 p.m., Mrs. Thompson is found without pulse or respiration, attempts at resuscitation were unsuccessful and she was pronounced dead at 5:27 p.m. Did you *cause* Mrs. Thompson's death.

- Were *damages* sustained?

B. Mr. Rodebush

Mr. Rodebush, who had Alzheimer's Disease, was a resident of the New Horizon Nursing Home. That morning Mr. Rodebush was taken by Nurse Aid John to the whirlpool bath at approximately 6:30 a.m. They were there about 30 minutes.

After the bath, John reported to Nurse Manager George that Mr. Rodebush had a "rash" on his face. John detected the smell of alcohol on John's breath. When asked about it, John admitted to George that he had partied all night and came directly to work from the party. George sent John home, which was at approximately 7:30 a.m. When Mrs. Rodebush arrived at New Horizon at about noon, she noticed large welts and red marks on her husband's face. She requested that Mr. Rodebush be examined by his physician. In the physician's opinion, the welts and marks were between 6 and 12 hours old and were caused by slaps of a human hand.

- Did Nurse Aid John owe a *duty* to Mr. Rodebush? Did he commit *malpractice* by breaching any duty? Was there *causation* of an injury? Did Mr. Rodebush sustain damages?

- What was Nurse Manager George's *duty* to Mr. Rodebush?

Mr. Rodebush brought a lawsuit against New Horizon allegedly: (1) negligence in hiring practices; (2) negligence in supervising John; and (3) intentional infliction of physical injury and emotional distress.

- Was New Horizon liable for the *intentional tort*, the slapping of Mr. Rodebush by Nurse Aid John?

- Was Nurse Manager George *negligent* in supervising John?

- Was John's conduct within the *scope of employment* for a nurse aid?

New Horizon was found to have violated the following policies: (1) background check not obtained; (2) no documentation of training or instruction provided to John; (3) failure to notify Ms. Rodebush of the injury; (4) failure to timely follow procedures of an intoxicated employee; (5) fail to have a licensed nurse on duty at time of the incident; and (6) fail to notify physician of the incident.

- Was the conduct of New Horizon and its employees' *willful misconduct*, wanton or reckless disregard for Mr. Rodebush?

SECTION 10-2: MISPLACED CENTRAL VENOUS LINE

Mrs. P was admitted to the hospital complaining of abdominal pain. After six days of testing, exploratory surgery was performed, in which the anesthesiologist inserted a central venous catheter line into Mrs. P's neck. The patient later complained of pain and was given an epidural, at which point her blood pressure dropped to critical levels. Dr. Surgeon, after reviewing x-rays of the catheter placement, supervised Dr. Resident who pulled the tip of the catheter back. Mrs. P's blood pressure remained low for almost three hours, at which time she suffered a cardiac arrest, resulting in profound brain damage.

Hospital policy required x-ray confirmation of central venous line placement within one hour of a patient leaving the operating room. Policy also required the on-duty radiologist to read the x-rays immediately and report the results to the patient's nurse. The x-rays were taken 30 minutes after the patient left the OR, which showed misplacement of the catheter into the right atrium of the patient's heart.

The nurses in the recovery room failed to document whether they had received x-ray confirmation of the catheter's placement or whether they took any follow-up action. They claimed that they used a peripheral line in Mrs. P's arm to insert IV fluids; however, they failed to document where and when they inserted the IV fluids. The radiologist failed to document whether he had read the x-rays or reported the results to the nurses.

SECTION 10-3: PROBLEMATIC LABOR AND DELIVERY

A. Birth of Baby Boy Y

Mrs. Y arrived at the hospital on July 28 at 0015 a.m. with a history of bleeding and contractions since midnight. The nurses notes indicate her EDC as July 14. Fetal heart tones were taken on admission by fetoscope and were 140. Mrs. Y's contractions were of moderate intensity and 3 minutes apart. On vaginal examination, she was 4cm dilated.

Mrs. Y was in labor for the next 7 hours. During the first two hours, the baby's heart tones were monitored by fetoscope. The medical record indicated that fetal heart tones were noted at 0035, 0105, 0130, 0145, and 0205. An external monitor was started at 0215. All the fetal heart tones taken were between 140 and 150. The external monitor ran for an hour and a half but the tape was not very good. Contractions on the tape were only shown intermittently, although the nurses indicated that Mrs. Y continued to have contractions 3 minutes apart with moderate intensity. At several places on the external monitor tape there were dips in the fetal heart tones without corresponding contractions. At 0345, the nurses removed the external monitor at the order of Dr. P, Mrs. Y's private physician, and continued fetal heart monitoring by fetoscope. The fetoscope readings were taken at 0348 and 0410, and were 120 at each reading.

At 0430, Dr. Resident arrived and attached an internal lead for an internal monitor. Mrs. Y was monitored internally from 0430 to 0445. During that time, her contractions were every 2-2 1/2 minutes apart and had intensified. The baseline of the fetal heart tones was 120, the variability poor, and the tape demonstrated late decelerations beginning at 0445. At 0500 and again at 0515 the nurses noticed several prolonged late decelerations. At 0530, Dr. Resident returned and checked on Mrs Y. Dr. Resident immediately called Dr. P, who arrived at 0615. Dr. P. ordered a stat C-Section at 0630; however, the baby was not delivered until 0730. The baby had Apgars of 0 and 3 at 1 and 5 minutes of life. CRNA provided anesthesia during delivery and noted that at birth Baby Boy Y was cyanotic and very flaccid, and that she aspirated the trachea, intubated and provided oxygen by positive pressure. At 3 minutes of life, Dr. Pediatrician, who happened to be in the hospital, arrived. He immediately extubated Baby Boy Y, aspirated the lungs, found thick meconium fluid, reintubated the baby, and supplied oxygen by positive pressure. At 10 minutes of life, Baby Boy Y had an Apgar of 6. Unfortunately, Baby Boy Y was diagnosed with cerebral palsy with severe mental retardation and spastic quadriplegia.

Additional verified facts:

1. The hospital had a policy that stated electronic fetal monitoring is not required during the active phase of labor provided heart tones are listened to by fetoscope every 15 minutes for 60 seconds duration and the results are charted.

2. If an external or internal monitor is used, the nurses must ascertain whether the monitor is accurately recording the baby's fetal heart tones as well as the mother's contractions.

3. Dr. Resident testified that he was in the hospital all night and could have been reached at any time by the nurses.

4. Dr. Resident testified that it wasn't until 0430 that he was alerted by the nurses that the external monitor was not picking up the mother's contractions, or that Mrs. Y may have been 6 weeks overdue and may have been bleeding for 24 hours.

5. When Dr. Resident notified Dr. P at 0530 and advised him about the prolonged late decelerations and suggested preparations be made for C-Section, Dr. P said to wait until he arrived; however, there was no documentation of this conversation.

6. Dr. P did not call a pediatrician because he felt this was the responsibility of either the labor and delivery nurses or the resident.

7. CRNA testified that although her operative note indicated that she aspirated the trachea, this meant that she had aspirated below the vocal chords and she had suctioned off as much of the meconium as possible, and after intubating the baby, she applied positive pressure oxygen by Ambu bag.

8. Mrs. Y told the nurse upon arrival at the hospital that she had been bleeding and cramping since midnight of the day before, and that her due date was the middle of June.

B. Birth of Baby Boy S

Mrs. S first sought prenatal care when 4 months pregnant. She was a smoker of $1^{1}/_{2}$ packs a day but had no other problems noted. During her 5th and 6th months, she failed to keep prenatal appointments. When she showed up at 34 weeks by dates with a fundal height of 30 weeks and no weight gain noted during her pregnancy, Dr. G. ordered an ultrasound exam, a NST, and biophysical profile. The ultrasound showed a BPD consistent with 30 weeks and the baby was active. Dr. G counseled Mrs. S about smoking and gave her an appointment with a dietician. Mrs. S failed to keep the appointment with the dietician.

Dr. G subsequently discharged Mrs. S as a patient due to non compliance. Mrs. S therefore showed up every few weeks in the emergency department of the hospital complaining of pains, was monitored and found not to be in labor, and sent home (with a doctor's appointment that she failed to keep).

On her due date, Mrs. S had SROM with thick meconium fluid. When she was admitted to labor and delivery, her blood pressure was 160/100. She was placed on an external monitor and the baby was active. The nurse commented to Mrs. S about the brand new monitors they were just trying out. A routine call was put in for a doctor who answered 15 minutes later. In the meantime, Mrs. S started contracting and the monitor tracing became unreadable. An internal lead was sought; however, it took about 30 minutes to locate the lead as Central Supply had just gotten them in. As she placed the lead, the nurse commented, "I didn't think they'd ever find it." Mrs. S was dilated sufficiently to place the internal lead. Late decelerations were noted. A second page for a doctor was placed, this time stat. Dr. C answered and requested set up for a C-Section. Mrs. S then screamed: "the baby's coming" and within 10 minutes delivered with Dr. C in attendance. In all of the excitement, the assigned pediatrician was not called until 10 minutes prior to delivery and missed it by 5 minutes.

Comments in the delivery room amid the confusion included: "Where is Dr. C? I paged her 10 minutes ago. Has anyone seen Dr. Pediatrician? I forgot to call him. We are so short-staffed today. Can you stay late again? If they don't get us more help. . . . Who knows how to work this thing? How do you turn this on? You've contaminated it!"

Baby Boy S delivered in a sea of green meconium and was suctioned by Dr. C. The infant is limp with a heart rate of 50 at 1 minute. The baby is bagged after suctioning and begins to respond with respiratory effort though he remains cyanotic. He is post-term, severely malnourished, weighs about 5 lbs, and

Apgars are 1 and 7. Baby Boy S is intubated and placed on a ventilator. At 6 hours of age seizures begin. During a seizure, the baby's oxygen monitor dropped. Mrs. S asked the respiratory therapist at the bedside if the oxygen level was OK, to which the respiratory therapist responded: "These monitors are always off, don't worry."

At the time of discharge, Dr. Pediatrician told Mrs. S the baby looked good. A follow-up appointment was made for two weeks but was not kept. Mrs. S took Baby Boy S to the Health Department for his shots. At 6 months of age he was slow in development. A lawsuit was filed at 1 year of age.

Issues to discuss:

1. Effects of smoking and Mrs. S's responsibility for those effects.
2. Mrs. S's responsibility for receiving and continuing prenatal care.
3. How does a doctor dismiss a patient from her practice?
4. What communication problems with the nurses in labor and delivery raise liability issues?
5. Identify key points of documentation and what would be particularly important to have documented.
6. Was there liability for the equipment? Whose liability?
7. How would you apportion fault?

SECTION 10-4: ETHICAL CHALLENGES

A. Clarence Higgins

Clarence Higgins, an elderly man in his eighties, was admitted to the hospital with shortness of breath due to an unknown cause. Mr. Higgins' wife died four years ago and since that time he has lived alone. He has been an active, alert person.

Mr. Higgins' physician, Dr. Spendlove, admitted him to a monitored bed and wrote in his admission orders that in the event of cardiac or respiratory arrest, Mr. Higgins was not to be subjected to chest compressions but he should receive medications.

Ten days after admission, Mr. Higgins had an episode of chest pain and palpitations (ventricular tachycardia) for about twenty seconds. Nurse Albright was alerted to this by the monitor and came immediately into his room and administered a precordial thump to his chest. This converted Mr. Higgins' cardiac rhythm back to normal. Mr. Higgins was upset by this episode and told Nurse Albright, "Don't you even do that to me again." Questioning clarified that Mr.

Higgins meant "I want to be allowed to die in peace." Nurse Albright recorded his remarks in the nurse's notes.

Nurse Albright realized it was Dr. Spendlove's day off, and knew from experience that Dr. Delbert, the on-call physician for Dr. Spendlove, would not alter her partner's orders. Therefore, Nurse Albright did not call Dr. Delbert to inform her of Mr. Higgins' wishes.

A few minutes later, Mr. Higgins told Nurse Albright that he wanted to talk to "the person responsible for living wills" to assure that he would not be subjected to a resuscitation attempt. A chaplain was called who met with Mr. Higgins about thirty minutes later. Mr. Higgins told her, "I want to die and be with my wife. I do not wish to be brought back if something serious goes wrong." A living will form was left with Mr. Higgins. These facts were reported to Nurse Albright.

Dr. Fenwick, a consulting physician, arrived on the floor around 2:00 p.m. She was asked for a DNR order for Mr. Higgins. She refused, saying she did not have the authority to write such an order.

At the 3:00 p.m. change of shift, Mr. Higgins said to the evening nurse, "I do not want anything done to me if anything happens." Nurse Richards reported this to Nurse Albright and the nursing director. However, no action was taken by any of these nurses. Nurse Richards conveyed all of this information to Nurse Clay, the night shift nurse who came on duty at 11:00 p.m.

At 3:00 a.m. the next morning, Mr. Higgins, who was asleep, began to have episodes of rapid heartbeat. The monitor showed this to be supra-ventricular tachycardia. These episodes continued until 3:45 a.m. with spontaneous resolution, and Mr. Higgins remained asleep throughout. At 4:30 a.m., Nurse Clay called Dr. Spendlove and told him about Mr. Higgins' episodes of supra-ventricular tachycardia.

At 5:45 a.m., Mr. Higgins' pulse stopped. The monitor showed a chaotic heartbeat (ventricular fibrillation). Mr. Higgins became unarousable and ceased breathing. The ventricular fibrillation was treated with medications per the CPR protocol and the orders written in Mr. Higgins' chart.

At 5:56 a.m., Dr. Spendlove was called and told that Mr. Higgins had been without respirations since 5:49. Dr. Spendlove was not told of Mr. Higgins' wishes regarding resuscitation. Dr. Spendlove ordered a full resuscitation attempt and CPR was begun.

B. Phyllis Lohmann

Phyllis Lohmann is a seventy-two year old woman with COPD. She is a widow with two adult children. In recent months, Mrs. Lohmann and her physician, Dr. Cranshaw, had discussed her condition and agreed that it would be reasonable for her to have a DNR order since it was unlikely, were her COPD to become exacerbated, for her to ever come off the ventilator. Mrs. Lohmann wrote an advance directive to this effect.

Mrs. Lohmann was admitted to the hospital yesterday morning with a distended abdomen and complaining of abdominal pain. Dr. Cranshaw ordered oxygen to be given by mask and wrote a DNR order in her chart after he spoke with her. A workup was ordered and consultants were called in.

By that evening, Nurse Perkins observed that Mrs. Lohmann was extremely diaphoretic, gray and dyspneic. Her abdomen was very large, firm and tender to touch. Although her pulse-oximetry was 58%-60%, Mrs. Lohmann was alert and oriented. She told Nurse Perkins that she wanted "everything done;" she wanted to be put on a ventilator if needed, but did not want to be kept on one for a prolonged period of time if she was going to be a "vegetable." Mrs. Lohmann repeated this statement in the presence of the charge nurse and team leader.

Dr. Anderson was on call for Dr. Cranshaw. When Nurse Perkins told Dr. Anderson about Mrs. Lohmann's condition and statements, Dr. Anderson ordered that Mrs. Lohmann not be put on the ventilator and not be given CPR. Nurse Perkins asked if arterial blood gases could be obtained. Dr. Anderson refused to order them. When told Mrs. Lohmann's oxygen saturation, Dr. Anderson said he did not want to be notified about them.

The nursing supervisor was called and told of the situation. She spoke with Mrs. Lohmann. It was evident to her that Mrs. Lohmann was in imminent danger of arrest if something was not done for her fairly soon. Following her conversation with Mrs. Lohmann, the nursing supervisor ordered that she be moved to the MICU and intubated.

C. Welby Collins

Welby Collins, a sixty-three year old man with a history of heart problems, had a major heart attack at home and was transferred from a small rural hospital near his home to another hospital some distance away. The transferring physician, Mr. Collins' personal physician, reported that Mr. Collins had a living will and had spoken to her of his wishes regarding life support. "Mr. Collins did not want life support prolonged if it was unreasonable to expect a good outcome with a full restoration of function."

On admission to the hospital, Mr. Collins was unable to speak for himself. He arrived intubated and was put in the cardiac intensive care unit. When Mrs. Collins was asked if her husband had a living will, she said, "yes," but chose not to have a copy put in his chart.

Dr. Tannen, the receiving physician, spoke with Mrs. Collins and her three adult children. Dr. Tannen thought that he could pull Mr. Collins through this episode and Mrs. Collins said she wanted "everything done."

Over the next ten days, Mr. Collins' condition steadily deteriorated and he did not regain the ability to speak for himself. His kidneys failed and he seemed to suffer a neurological injury, perhaps due to a stroke, such that his right side was flaccid. Dr. Tannen continued to hold out hope to the Collins' family and they continued to insist that full supportive care be given.

To the nurses caring for Mr. Collins it seemed that, in the unlikely event Mr. Collins survived his illness, he would most likely suffer permanent neurological and physiological deficits.

Mr. Collins' family seemed locked in denial. It was also common knowledge in the hospital that Dr. Tannen's father was terminally ill with cancer and that he was having difficulty dealing with his father's illness.

D. Thelma Winkler

Thelma Winkler is a fifty-four year old woman with a long history of severe asthma. She and her husband, Willie, live in a neighboring state. They were visiting relatives here when Thelma suffered an asthma attack in the middle of the night. This awakened Willie. Thelma, as was her custom, gathered her inhalants and left the room so as to not disturb her husband. Willie knew that Thelma would not want him hovering so he stayed in their room, but he did not go back to sleep. About fifteen minutes later, Willie went to check on Thelma and found her without pulse or respirations. Willie called 911 and began CPR.

Thelma has been in intensive care for five weeks now. She has never regained consciousness and has no responses, except to deep pain. The neurologist has told Willie and their two adult daughters that chances for a good neurological recovery are poor.

The family has told the nursing staff that Thelma had never wanted to be fussed over. She did not allow her asthma to keep her from being active in civic clubs and in the children's school activities. She usually doctored herself rather than go to a physician. Thelma did not like to talk about her illness. When family members would speak of their own wishes regarding life support in the event of serious illness, Thelma refused to join in the conversation and would usually leave the room. Thus, Thelma had no advance directive for health care. Willie and his daughters tell the nurses that they do not think Thelma would want treatment to continue in these circumstances.

Thelma's attending physician, Dr. Robard, visits with her family only briefly and gives reports on the progress of her lungs and kidneys. He expects her to be able to be eventually weaned from the ventilator. The family has told Dr. Robard that they do not think Thelma would want treatment continued.

E. Mary Long

Mary Long is an eighty-two year old woman who was living by herself at her apartment until she was found on the floor by her neighbor, unconscious and unable to move her right side. After being admitted to the hospital, a CT scan of her brain showed a new ischemic infarction (stroke) to account for her weakness but also many other old infarctions.

Mrs. Long had not been followed on a regular basis by a physician. She had a history of hypertension but had refused to take medications for this over the last one to two years. She had been admitted to the hospital two years ago for a stroke resulting in mild residual weakness but had cognitive loss noted then.

Mrs. Long is a widow who has two children, one daughter living near her and one son in Arizona. She has no other relatives. Her neighbor, a nurse, and also her only friend, looked in on her every day and would buy groceries for her. The neighbor noted that for the last two years, Mrs. Long had had progressive loss in memory and other cognitive functions, had more problems with balance and speech, and rarely left her apartment. She had an unkempt apartment and had to be encouraged to bathe. The apartment manager had frequently threatened to evict Mrs. Long but the neighbor was able to keep her and the apartment acceptably clean. Mrs. Long was incontinent of urine and occasionally incontinent of stool.

The symptoms from the stroke improved somewhat over the next two weeks as Mrs. Long became more alert. She still could not communicate effectively to comprehend or help in decisionmaking as her speech and cognitive skills were severely limited. She was able to sit in a chair but needed two people to transfer her. She was unable to feed herself and when handfed, she would hold the food in her mouth and rarely would swallow, despite intensive speech therapy and nursing. She was receiving IV fluids during this period. She did not appear to recognize her daughter but appeared to recognize her neighbor.

As her nutritional status was quite poor and oral feedings became inadequate to maintain life, the attending physician sought additional help in determining her prognosis. Due to her progressive history of multiple infarct dementia, and after ruling out other treatable causes of dementia, the consulting and attending physicians felt that Mrs. Long may regain more function over the next one to two months but never be able to live by herself, communicate effectively, make decisions for herself, or walk or transfer by herself. She would need to have total care supplied by someone else and be at high risk for developing decubitus ulcers, aspiration pneumonia, and other complications from immobility. Knowing the prognosis, the attending physician discussed with the daughter and neighbor the concerns over the appropriateness of artificial nutrition.

Mrs. Long had evidently discussed her wishes about medical care decisions with her neighbor frequently over the last four years. She stated she would not want any type of life support, including a feeding tube, if she could not be independent and care for herself. She stated that she would rather die than live in a nursing home. While Mrs. Long still had capacity, the neighbor had her fill out an advance directive with additional instructions addressing these wishes.

The daughter, who was alienated from her mother, would occasionally call the neighbor and see how she was doing and then report this to her brother in Arizona. The daughter had, however, not spoken to her mother in the last four to five years. The son had written on a routine basis to his mother in the past, but over the last four years he had stopped writing as she had not responded to his letters. He had not visited her in four years.

Although the son and neighbor agree that Mrs. Long would not want an artificial feeding tube placed, the daughter disagrees and refuses to let her mother "starve to death."

F. Betty Boyd

Betty Boyd was diagnosed as having first stage Alzheimer's disease in 1988 shortly after the death of her husband. Occasionally she was discovered lost in her own neighborhood and uncertain about the day, time or month. She was periodically uncertain about her own surroundings. This panicked her, her family, and neighbors. She was, however, emphatic about the desire to stay in her own home, saying, "I always lived there with my husband and I want to stay there."

As the Alzheimer's disease progressed, Mrs. Boyd became less and less capable of any care for herself. At this time, her family initiated discussions in her lucid moments about her wishes for future treatment after having come to grips with the Alzheimer's disease and with the problems that would arise. However, whenever discussions were raised, Mrs. Boyd greeted the remarks with absolute silence, or simply stated that she wanted to live if it was possible for her to remember. Her lucid moments became less and less and she required more and more care by her family. Her financial resources were exhausted and her children became more tired of caring for her.

In 1990, other medical problems began. In that year, Mrs. Boyd fell and broke a hip. This led to serious questions about her need for twenty-four hour supervision. This required the family to make a decision as to whether to keep her in their home and find people to come in and care for her during the day, use the services of an adult day care center in the neighborhood, or to institutionalize her in an intermediate care nursing home. The family decided to keep her at home and use both the adult day care center and some of their resources to hire live-in help on days when the day care center was not feasible.

In 1991, still other problems arose. Mrs. Boyd was diagnosed as having diabetes. Also that year, she contracted pneumonia and suffered congestive heart failure. Each time Mrs. Boyd was brought to the hospital, increasing numbers of questions were asked about how serious the disease was, how aggressive they should be in treating her, and what were the best options available for her care. With each passing disease, Mrs. Boyd became less and less capable of participating in any decisions. Finally, the decision was made to transfer her to a long-term care facility.

In this facility, the ability to perform CPR was limited. A question was raised as to whether Mrs. Boyd should have a do not resuscitate order written if she should experience acute cardiac failure. The family could not agree whether this should be done. Questions were also raised about whether Mrs. Boyd should be transferred to an acute care hospital should other medical complications arise. Some of the family increasingly felt that she should be left in the long-term care facility to die. However, her physician and the institution encouraged treatment of any problem that would be easily cured.

In June 1992, Mrs. Boyd had a small stroke and lost most of her spontaneous movements on her left side and became totally noncommunicative. Questions were raised as to whether she could swallow safely and whether a feeding tube should be used. The physician suggested that a feeding tube be inserted to minimize the possibility of her aspirating food into her lungs or choking on food when she ate. While some of the family agreed with this, others objected strenuously. Eventually the institution and the physician prevailed and Mrs. Boyd was force fed.

On April 5, 1992, Mrs. Boyd exhibited symptoms of acute respiratory distress. Hospitalization was requested by the skilled nursing facility and the physician. They felt that the acute respiratory distress could be overcome and that Mrs. Boyd would be able to return to the skilled nursing facility. Some of the family questioned the hospitalization but were ultimately forced into it.

At the hospital, it was discovered that Mrs. Boyd had an exceptionally low white blood count. The physician feared what would happen if an infection should set in given the respiratory distress. The physician recommended a blood transfusion. The respiratory stridor also puzzled the physician and he suggested a bronchoscopy. In both cases again the family was in conflict. The physician thus continued aggressive treatment on Mrs. Boyd.

SECTION 10-5: DELAYED DIAGNOSIS OF NEWBORN INFECTION

Baby Girl X was born at 11:20 at the hospital. There was a vacuum extraction, but birth was not difficult. Baby Girl X had Apgar scores of 8 at 1 minutes and 9 at 5 minutes. At 1400, Baby Girl X was brought to her mother's room. At this point, she seemed normal; heart and respiratory rates were unremarkable. At 1600, a nurse came into the mom's room. The mom spoke only Spanish; the was no nurse on duty who understood Spanish. However, the mom's bilingual 15 year old niece was present and told the nurse that Baby Girl X would not suck, was irritable and crying. The nurse commented that the baby's head was probably sore due to the vacuum extraction. The nurse did not exam Baby Girl X. At 1900, friends visited; one told the nurse Baby Girl X would not feed. Again, the nurse did not come into the room and examine the infant.

From 1600 to 2300, Baby Girl X was making slight grunts on expiration and still would not feed. At 2300, the nurse came into the room and assessed the infant. The nursing record stated: "On and off grunting; mottling of lower extremities. Temperature 100.7."

At 2330, the nurse called Dr. Pediatrician. This was the first time he had been notified of the baby's birth. The nurse told Dr. Pediatrician the baby was "slightly jaundiced" and there was "on and off fast breathing." The nurse did not tell Dr. Pediatrician of the slight grunting with expiration or the mottling of the lower limbs. Dr. Pediatrician ordered a complete blood count and told the nurse, "call me if the child is worse." Dr. Pediatrician called back at 0030 and was told by the nurse there was increased mottling with off and on grunting respirations. Dr. Pediatrician instructed the nurse to immediately contact Dr. Neonatologist and send the baby to the NICU. The nurse called Dr. Neonatologist at 0045. He ordered a complete infection workup and told the nurse to administer antibiotics. Dr. Neonatologist arrived at the hospital at 0155; however, at 0120 Baby Girl X has severe seizures.

At 0210, Baby Girl X was given antibiotics. A diagnosis of Group B Streptococcus Meningitis was made. Baby Girl X had a stormy course; she has severe residual brain damage with spastic quadriplegia and cortical blindness, and will require medical and attendant care for life.

SECTION 10-6: ALTERED AND LOST MEDICAL RECORDS

In 1987, Mrs. Mosk has a tumor removed from her left leg by Dr. Surgeon, which was found to be benign. In 1994, Dr. Surgeon removed a second mass from Mrs. Mosk's leg. This mass was a low-grade malignant dermatofibrosarcoma protuberans.

In 1995, Mrs. Mosk developed degenerative arthritis in her knees and had surgery by Dr. Rheumatologist in October 1995 and again in May 1996, replacing Mrs. Mosk's knee joints. After surgery, Mrs. Mosk visited Dr. Rheumatologist's office a number of times and was frequently seen by APN Mary. On October 2, 1996, Mrs. Mosk saw APN Mary and complained of a lump on her leg. APN Mary examined Mrs. Mosk and detected a "small calcified lesion along the Achilles tendon." APN Mary did not have Mrs. Mosk see Dr. Rheumatologist nor did APN Mary recommend a biopsy of the lesion. APN Mary reassured Mrs. Mosk that nothing was wrong although APN Mary was aware of the previous tumors.

On November 3, 1996, Mrs. Mosk was admitted to hospital for a right knee revision by Dr. Rheumatologist. Prior to surgery, Mrs. Mosk was examined by an RN who documented in her hospital medical record the existence of a "firm nodule measuring 1cm by 1cm" on Mrs. Mosk's left Achilles tendon. However, the RN did not specifically tell Dr. Rheumatologist or APN Mary about the lesion.

Following surgery, Mrs. Mosk continued to see Dr. Rheumatologist and APN Mary. On November 10, 1997 (approximately 1 year later), Dr. Rheumatologist removed the mass from Mrs. Mosk's left leg. The tumor had more than doubled in size since November 1996 and was diagnosed as an epithelioid carcinoma, a rare form of malignant soft tissue cancer. A bone scan revealed that the cancer had metastasized to Mrs. Mosk's shoulder and right femur. Dr. Rheumatologist referred Mrs .Mosk to Dr. Orthopod. Dr. Orthopod was sent Mrs. Mosk's original medical record from Dr. Rheumatologist's office, consisting of 7 pages of notes.

In December 1997, Dr. Orthopod was requested to return to Dr. Rheumatologist the original office medical record for Mrs. Mosk. In January 1998, Dr. Orthopod was again requested to return the original medical record for Mrs. Mosk from Dr. Rheumatologist's office. However, at this time it was discovered that the original medical record had vanished.

Facts:

1. When Dr. Orthopod was deposed, he had a copy of page 7 from Dr. Rheumatologist's office medical record for Mrs. Mosk. There was a type written entry dated September 21, 1997: "Mrs. Mosk comes in today for her evaluation on the radiographs reviewed with radiologist. Radiologist not impressed that mass on left leg anything other than a benign problem, perhaps fibroma. Will continue to observe."

2. When Dr. Rheumatologist was deposed he produced a *copy* of his office record for Mrs. Mosk. On Dr. Rheumatologist's copy, the September 21, 1997 entry did not contain this statement, "Will con-

tinue to observe." However, it included a handwritten notation by Dr. Rheumatologist: "As she does not want excisional biopsy, we will observe."

3. Dr. Rheumatologist testified that he did not know about the mass on the left Achilles tendon until February 26, 1997.

4. Office notebooks with telephone messages received from Mrs. Mosk reflected:

   - February 26, 1997—Secretary's entry: "Mosk, right foot, coming in today." Dr. Rheumatologist penciled in notation: "Patient seen, refuses workup, left foot, workup left foot."

   - May 5, 1997—Secretary's entry: "Mrs. Mosk called and complaining of pain in her left leg." Dr. Rheumatologist penciled in notation: "Mrs. Mosk refuses to have tumor biopsied."

   - September 11, 1997—Secretary's entry "Mrs. Mosk called complaining of the lump on her left leg." Dr. Rheumatologist penciled in notation: "Today Mrs. Mosk has agreed to a workup." (This contradicts the handwritten notation by Dr. Rheumatologist in his September 21, 1997 entry in his copy of Mrs. Mosk's medical record."

5. At trial, expert witness for Mrs. Mosk testified that had the tumor been removed by March 1997, the cancer would not have metastasized and Mrs. Mosk would have fully recovered. By the time of trial, Mrs. Mosk had died.

SECTION 10-7: SALES REP IN OR
Facts:

1. Following a routine outpatient removal of a benign fibroid tumor in her uterus, 30 year old woman died of cardiac arrest.

2. One of the doctors performing the surgery was on 5 years probation for professional misconduct.

3. Both physicians performing the surgery were unfamiliar with and unauthorized to use the equipment causing the death, a new Bipolar Hysteroscopy Electrosurgery System.

4. The Electrosurgery System had not been approved by the hospital; however, the sales representative rolled it into the hospital on the day of surgery.

5. The physicians and nurses had no formal training in use of the Electrosurgery System.

6. Patient was never given the chance to consent to the use of the new Electrosurgery System or the presence of the sales rep in the OR.

7. The operating room nurses expressed concern to the physicians that they were not trained in assisting with the new equipment; the physicians dismissed their concerns and told them not to worry because the sale representative would operate the controls, a violation of hospital policy.

8. The nurses failed to report the intent of the sales rep to operate the equipment to their supervisors and failed to refuse the improper physicians' orders.

9. During the surgery, a nurse noticed that the fluid was not properly draining; when she told the surgeons, they said not to worry.

SECTION 10-8: DUTY TO EMERGENCY DEPARTMENT PATIENT

Sally presents to the Outpatient Department at Community Hospital, threatening suicide. Community Hospital does not have a psychiatrist or psychologist on its Medical Staff, nor does it offer behavioral health services. The registration clerk in the Outpatient Department realizes that Sally needs medical services that Community Hospital doesn't have. The registration clerk tells Sally to go to the Emergency Department.

The ED physician examines Sally, determines that she is medically stable, but diagnoses her as suicidal. The ED nurse is requested to contact Medical Center, which has behavioral health services available. The ED nurse contacts Medical Center, is told that a bed is available on its behavioral health unit, and is instructed that he will need to contact the psychiatrist on call at the Medical Center to accept transfer of the patient.

The psychiatrist on-call at the Medical Center, Dr. Barb, tells the ED nurse that Sally is a former patient of hers, but she has terminated her relationship with Sally because she is non-compliant with treatment and sees multiple physicians to obtain medications. Dr. Barb therefore refuses to accept Sally as a patient.

SECTION 10-9: FLOATING

RN Jack arrives at Memorial General Hospital for his regular shift in the ICU. Due to a shortage of staff, RN Jack is told to float to the Orthopedics Unit and act as the Charge Nurse there. RN Jack refuses to accept the assignment because "he is unfamiliar with the Orthopedics Unit" and "feels incompetent to be there."

At Memorial General Hospital, floating is an established policy of which RN Jack was aware at that time of employment. RN Jack refused the assignment and was suspended without pay for two days.

When RN Jack returned to Memorial General Hospital, he told the Director of Nursing that he would not float "if he felt incompetent to do so." RN Jack was terminated by Memorial General Hospital and RN Jack sued.

Some of the issues:

- Was RN Jack "incompetent" to be assigned to the Orthopedic Unit?

- Was RN Jack "incompetent" to be the Charge Nurse on the Orthopedic Unit?

- Is floating an important public policy for hospitals?

- Should RN Jack win his lawsuit against the hospital?

SECTION 10-10: HOME HEALTH DILEMMAS

A. What Should Be Done With Mrs. K?

Mrs. K is 64 years old, divorced, and lives alone. She had MS and morbid obesity. She has a catheter. Although she has a Hoyer Lift, she refuses to get out of bed. Her perineal area and buttocks frequently break down, requiring aggressive care.

Mrs. K has two daughters who are alienated from their mother. No other family members are present. There is no apparent remaining social support for her. The daughters want Mrs. K to go to a nursing home.

Mrs. K is provided home maker services daily through the Division on Aging. She is assisted each day with her morning care and is provided meals. Mrs. K has a small refrigerator and microwave at her bedside. Care givers change frequently as "the patient is manipulative and difficult to please." Originally, the home health nurses saw Mrs. K on a daily basis to care for her tissue breakdown. As her condition improved, home health nurses saw her every other day. When she healed, home health nurses visited only one time per week. However, because of Mrs. K's immobility and her poor hygiene, tissue breakdown is a recurring problem.

Home health nurses have advised Mrs. K repeatedly of the need to hire more care as her needs aren't being met. Mrs. K has the financial resources to do so but refuses to consider hiring help. She spends large sums of money

245

repairing and redecorating her house but says "she can't afford to hire help." The home health nurses believe that Mrs. K is manipulating the system in terms of utilizing insurance, Medicare, and Medicaid benefits.

B. Mr. Walker and His Bride

Home Health Agency was contacted by Mr. Walker who is very ill with COPD. Mr. Walker is a man of stature in the community and can clearly afford Home Health Services. At the first interview, he tells you that "money is no object" and that his main goal is to stay at home. Although he is very sick and has been bed-bound for some time, he is a "newlywed and wants to be home with his bride." He tells you that he wants 24 hour care, i.e., 2 RNs for the day and an LPN at night.

After several weeks, the Home Health nurses begin to express concern about Mrs. Walker. Mrs. Walker is a heavy drinker and is jealous of the nurses. Mr. Walker's adult children also have concerns about Mrs. Walker. They tell the Home Health nurses that they believe Mrs. Walker is abusive to Mr. Walker. They ask you if there is any evidence that their suspicions are founded, and whether Mrs. Walker should be hotlined for adult abuse and neglect.

The Home Health nurses are concerned about what it going on between Mr. and Mrs. Walker. Mrs. Walker insists that the Home Health nurses do not enter their bedroom unless she specifically asks them to. Often the sound of angry exchanges come from their bedroom. Once a nurse heard what she thought was Mr. Walker falling, and severe bruises were noticed. When asked what happened, Mr. Walker would not discuss it, and Mrs. Walker said that he had fallen when she tried to help him "to his favorite chair by the window." In addition, Mr. Walker has a foley catheter and after time alone in their bedroom, Mr. Walker frequently has blood in his urine. Urinary tract infections have also been a chronic problem.

On another occasion, Mr. Walker choked and his wife tried to prevent the Home Health nurse from calling 911.

Because Mrs. Walker becomes so angry when she reads anything not to her liking in her husband's medical records, the nurses are keeping double records.

C. Who Advocates for the Patient?

Karen is a 36 year old mother of two small children. She has severely debilitating MS but is able to remain in her home with extensive help from the Home Health Agency and volunteer friends. Karen is now unable to swallow food or water safely. She had lost weight to the point of life threatening malnutrition. By carefully listening to her indistinct speech at a family conference, all members of her family clearly understood that she did not want a gastric feeding tube or

IV tube for feeding or hydration. Karen said, "I have suffered so long that I am ready to die." The family tried in vain to change her mind.

Karen's "family" consists of her mother, step-father, and a sister. An insurance policy of $150,000, with the estranged father of her second child as the beneficiary, is the center of attention. The family has unsuccessfully persuaded Karen to change the policy and name one of them as the beneficiary. Karen believes that the father of the child will use the money to benefit both children.

The family took Karen to her neurologist, who sees her at infrequent intervals. According to the neurologist note, "After much conversation, the patient finally agreed to the gastric tube." Karen is now in a long-term care facility receiving nutrition and hydration through a gastric tube.

REFERENCES

American Nurses Association, *Implementing Nursing's Report Card: A Study of RN Staffing, Length of Stay, and Patient Outcomes.* American Nurses Publishing (1997).

Bauer, J. C., *Rural America and the Digital Transformation of Health Care*, 23 Journal of Legal Medicine 73 (March 2002).

Berg, J. W., *Ethics and E-Medicine*, 46 St. Louis University Law Journal 61 (Winter 2002).

Blegen, M. A., et al., *Nursing Staffing and Patient Outcomes*, 47 Nursing Research, 43 (1998).

Cardwell, M. S. *Interhospital Transfers of Obstetric Patients Under the Emergency Medical Treatment and Active Labor Act*, 16 The Journal of Legal Medicine 357 (1995).

Dimoff, J. C., *The Inadequacy of the IDEA in Assessing Mental Health for Adolescents: A Call for School-Based Mental Health,* 6 DePaul Journal of Health Care Law 319 (Spring 2003).

Doescher, M. P,. et al., *Racial and Ethical Disparities in Perceptions of Physician Style and Trust,* 9 Archives Fam. Med. 1156 (2000) (Lack of continuity in care has a greater impact than race or ethnicity).

Erdman, C., *The Medicolegal Dangers of Telephone Triage in Mental Health Care*, 22 Journal of Legal Medicine 553 (December 2001).

Furrow, B. R. *An Overview and Analysis of the Impact of the Emergency Medical Treatment and Active Labor Act,* 16 The Journal of Legal Medicine 325 (1995).

Gerberry, R. A., *Legal Ramifications of the Formation of Digital Hospitals,* 14 Health Lawyer 27 (June 2002).

Goodwin, A. B., *Striving For A Secure Environment: A Closer Look at Hospital Security Issues Following the Infant Abduction at Loyola University Medical Center,* 10 Annals of Health Law 245 (2001).

Granot, T. and Tabak, N., *Nursing Student's Right to Refuse to Treat Patients and the Relationship Between Year of Study and Attitude Towards Patient Care,* 21 Medicine and Law 549 (2002).

Hayley, D. C., et al., *Ethical and Legal Issues in Nursing Home Care,* 156 Archives of Internal Medicine 249 (Feb. 12, 1996).

Hogue, E. E., *Termination of Services: Legal Pitfalls for Home Health Care Providers,* 7 Journal of Home Health Care Practice 39 (1995).

Hospital Morality In Relation To Staff Workload: A Four-Year Study In An Adult Intensive Care Unit. 356 The Lancet, 185 (July 15, 2000).

Johns, J. A., *A Concept Analysis of Trust,* 76 J. Advanced Nursing (1996).

Kinsella, A., *Home Telehealthcare: An Idea Whose Time Has Come-But With Safety Concerns,* 19 Medical Malpractice Law 7 (May 2002).

Kovner, C. and Gergen, P. J. *Nursing Staffing Levels and Adverse Events Following Surgery In US Hospitals,* 30 Image: Journal of Nursing Scholarship 315 (1998).

LaZarus, J. B. and Downing, B. (Wendy), *Monitoring and Investigating Certified Registered Nurse Practitioner in Pain Management,* 31 Journal of Law, Medicine and Ethics 101 (Spring 2003).

Lehr, D. G. and Greene, J., *Educating Students with Complex Health Care Needs in Public Schools: The Intersection of Health Care, Education and the Law,* 5 Journal of Health Care Law and Policy 68 (2002).

Lewis, C. *Malpractice: The Damning Evidence Is Under Your Nose,* Medical Economics 229 (April 15, 1996).

Lewis, M. A., *Testing Students For Pregnancy: How Far Will the Courts Allow Schools to Go?* 33 McGeorge Law Review 155 (2001).

Mannino, K. M., *The Nursing Shortage: Contributing Factors, Risk Implications, and Legislative Efforts to Combat the Shortage,* 15 Loyola Consumer Law Review 143 92003).

Marshall, B. K., *Resident Safety and Medical Errors in Nursing Homes,* 24 Journal of Legal Medicine 51 (March 2003).

Menenberg, S. R., *Standard of Care in Documentation of Psychiatric Nursing Care,* 9 Clinical Nurse Specialist 140 (1995).

Nurse Staffing and Patient Outcomes In the Inpatient Hospital Setting. American Nurses Association (2000).

Phan, J. N., *The Graying of America: Protecting Nursing Home Residents by Allowing Regulatory and Criminal Statutes to Establish Standards of Care in Private Negligence Actions*, 2 Houston Journal of Health Law and Policy 297 (2002).

Schmidt, L. E., *The Legal Landscape for Advanced Practice Nurses: The Nurses Perspective,* 90 Illinois Bar Journal 485 (September 2002).

Schroedel, J. R. and Fiber, P., *Punitive Versus Public Health Oriented Responses to Drug Use By Pregnant Women*, 1 Yale Journal of Health Policy, Law & Ethics 217 (Spring 2001).

Schwab, N. C. and Gelfman, M. G. B. (editors), *Legal Issues in School Health Services: A Resource For School Administrators, School Attorneys, and School Nurses* (2001).

Scott, E. J., *Punitive Damages in Lawsuits Against Nursing Homes*, 23 Journal of Legal Medicine 115 (March 2002).

The Hospital Workforce Shortage: Immediate and Future. American Hospital Association (June 2001).

Wakefield, M., *Patient Safety and Medical Errors: Implications For Rural Health Care*, 23 Journal of Legal Medicine 43 (March 2002).

249

CHAPTER 11

Glossary of Terms
by Jim Coulter, R.N., B.S.N.[1]

Accreditation: An official authorization providing credentials for maintaining standards of professional practice and assuring quality care.

Administrative Agency: Governmental body that is not a legislative, executive, or judicial unit.

Administrative Law: Laws governing the activities and procedures used by administrative agencies.

Admissibility (in evidence): Evidence that may be properly introduced in a legal proceeding. The determination as to admissibility is based on legal rules of evidence and is made by the trial judge or a screening panel.

Admissions: Statements by a party that are admissible in evidence as an exception to the hearsay rule. In a malpractice proceeding, an admission would typically be a statement of culpability by the defendant.

Advance Directive: Mechanism to allow individuals, while still competent, to make known their decisions regarding health care treatment that may be required in the future.

Affidavit: Voluntary, written statement of facts made under oath before an officer of the court or before a notary public.

---

1 Jim Coulter, RN, BSN graduated from the University of Missouri at Kansas City with a Bachelor of Science Degree in Biology and from Rockhurst University with a Bachelor of Science in Nursing. Jim is currently a Health Law Analyst for Shughart Thomson & Kilroy in Kansas City, Missouri, and a clinical research nurse for a contract research organization in Lenexa, Kansas.

Allegation: Assertions of facts which may or may not be supportable by evidence; plaintiff's statement which he or she hopes to prove in a legal action.

Americans with Disabilities Act (ADA): Federal legislation of 1999 that prohibits discrimination on the basis of physical or mental disabilities and mandates affirmative action to remove obstacles that hamper disabled persons. It guarantees equal opportunities for individuals with disabilities in public accommodations, employment, transportation, state and local government, and telecommunications.

Answer: A legal document that contains a defendant's written response to a complaint or declaration in a legal proceeding. The answer typically either denies the allegations of the plaintiff or makes allegations as to why the plaintiff should not recover.

Appeal: The process by which a decision of a lower court is brought for review to a court of higher jurisdiction, typically known as an appellate court.

Appellant: Party bringing an appeal of a case to a higher court.

Appellate Court: The court that reviews trial court decisions. Appellate courts review the transcript of the trial court proceedings and determine whether there were errors of law committed by the trial court.

Appellee: Party defending an appeal of a case to a higher court.

Attorney at Law: Person who acts for someone else in legal matters.

Attorney-Client Privilege: The privilege under law that protects the information given to the attorney in confidence by the client. The attorney cannot be compelled to testify regarding privileged information.

Battery: The unauthorized touching of another.

Brain Death: When respiration and circulation are artificially maintained, and there is a total and irreversible cessation of all brain function, including the brain stem and that such determination is made by a licensed physician.

Burden of Proof: The necessity or duty of affirmatively proving a fact or facts in dispute. The plaintiff typically has the burden of proof.

Business Associate: On behalf of a covered entity, performs or assists in the performance of:

- Function or activity involving the use or disclosure of individually identifiable health information; or

- Provides legal, actuarial, accounting, consulting, data aggregation, management, administrative, accreditation or financial services to or for the covered entity which involves disclosure of individually identifiable health information.

Case: An action or cause of action; a matter in dispute; a lawsuit.

Case Law: Legal principles derived from judicial decisions. Case law differs from statutes, which are enacted by legislators, and regulations which are promulgated by governmental agencies.

Cause of Action: A set of alleged facts that a plaintiff uses to seek legal redress.

Claims-Made Insurance: Insurance covering lawsuits filed or claims made during the term of the policy.

Claims-Made Policy: Requires that the claim be submitted during the actual policy period.

Clerk of the Court: The person who is responsible for the administrative functions of the court.

Common Law: That body of law that was passed down to the colonies by the British legal system and has been interpreted and refined by case law.

Comparative Negligence/Contributory Negligence: Affirmative defenses, one or the other of which is recognized in all jurisdictions.

- *Comparative Negligence:* an affirmative defense that compares the negligence of the defendant to that of the plaintiff. The plaintiff may recover damages from a negligent defendant even if the plaintiff and defendant are equally at fault. It is only when the plaintiff's negligence is greater than the defendant's that there can be no recovery. The plaintiff's damages are reduced, however, by the percentage that her/his own fault contributed to the overall damage.

- *Contributory Negligence:* an affirmative defense that prevents recovery against a defendant when the plaintiff's own negligence contributed to his or her own injury, even though the defendant's negligence may also have contributed to the injury.

Complaint or Petition: A legal document that is the initial pleading on the part of the plaintiff in a civil lawsuit. The purpose of this document is to give the defendant notice of the alleged facts constituting the cause of action. The complaint is usually attached to the summons.

253

Contempt: Willful disobedience to or open disrespect for the rules or orders by a court or legislative body.

Contributory or Comparative Negligence: Two or more parties failed to perform at the appropriate standard. Each party has some degree of negligence in the error or malpractice.

Corporate Liability: Hospitals and their governing bodies may be held liable for injuries resulting from imprudent or careless supervision of members of their medical staffs.

Counterclaim: A claim presented by a defendant in opposition to or deduction from the claim of the plaintiff. A claim made by the defendant against the plaintiff in the same action.

Court Order: Direction of a court or judge made or entered in writing with which one must comply or risk a contempt action.

Court Trial: A trial without a jury, wherein a judge determines the facts as well as the law.

Covered Entity: a health plan, health care clearing house, or a health care provider.

Credentialing: A system based on accepted standard criteria for determining the competence and capabilities of a professional to provide quality care and to minimize risks.

Cross-examination: Questioning of a witness by the party opposed to the party who produces the witness.

Damages: The sum of money a court or jury awards as compensation for a tort. The law recognizes certain categories of damages. These categories are often imprecise and inconsistent. Variations exist among jurisdictions, and all are not strictly adhered to by the courts. The major categories are general, special, and punitive/exemplary damages.

- *General damages:* typically intangible damages, such as pain and suffering, disfigurement, interference with ordinary enjoyment of life, etc.

- *Special damages:* out of pocket damages, such as medical expenses, lost wages, rehabilitation, etc.

- *Punitive/exemplary damages:* damages awarded to the plaintiff in cases of intentional tort or gross negligence to punish the defendant or act as a deterrent to others.

Decedent: Deceased person.

Decision: Judgment or decree of a court.

Defendant: The individual or individuals who are sued by the plaintiff. The originally named defendants may add other defendants to the suit. Medical malpractice or professional negligence cases usually include multiple defendants.

De-Identification Of Protected Health Information: By removing specific information from the records, there is a very small risk that individual could be identified. The HIPAA regulations identify the following specific pieces of information that relate to the individual, relatives, household members, and employer that must be deleted prior to disclosure for the record set to be considered de-identified: names; address; all dates directly related to individual (birth, admission, discharge, death); telephone numbers; fax numbers; email address; Social Security number; medical number; health plan beneficiary number; account number; certificate/license number; vehicle identifier, serial number, license plate; device identifiers and serial numbers; Wed Universal Resource Locators (URLs); Internet Protocol (IP) address number; biometric identifiers (finger/voice prints); full face photographic or comparable image; and any other unique identifying number, characteristic, code.

Deposition:

- The testimony of a witness taken under oath but not in open court, as provided by court order or rule, reduced to writing and duly authenticated, and may be used in a trial of an action in court. It is sometimes used as synonymous with "affidavit" or "oath", but its technical meaning does not include such terms.

- A written declaration under oath, made upon notice to the adverse party for the purpose of enabling him to attend and be examined; or upon written interrogatories. The term sometimes is used in a special sense to denote a statement made orally by a person on oath before an examiner, commissioner, or officer of the court, (but not in open court), and taken down in writing by the examiner or under his direction.

Directed Verdict: A decision and order by the trial court by which the judge determines that a claim or defense lacks sufficient support in the evidence to let the claim or defense go to the jury for consideration. A directed verdict is usually granted against the party who has the burden of proof. It may be directed in favor of a party who has the burden of proof only if the evidence is conclusively in his favor. Judgment will be entered by the clerk according to the directed verdict.

Discovery: Pretrial procedures to learn of evidence to minimize the element of surprise at the time of trial. These typically include interrogatories and depositions but can also include requests for admission of facts and requests for documents.

Discovery Statute: Refers to a particular type of statute of limitations; the time period does not begin until the patient discovers the harm. For example, a foreign object left in a patient after surgery may not be discovered until years after the surgery; it is only after the discovery that the time period for the statute of limitations begins.

Designated Records Set: A group of records that includes: medical records; billing records; enrollment, payment, claims adjudication records; and case management records.

Dismissal: A legal denial. To dismiss a motion is to deny it; to dismiss an appeal is to affirm the judgment of the trial court.

Dismissal With Prejudice: An adjudication on the merits, and final disposition, barring the right to bring or maintain an action on the same claim or cause.

Dismissal Without Prejudice: Dismissal without prejudice to the right of the complainant to sue again on the same cause of action. The effect of the words "without prejudice" is to prevent the decree of dismissal from operating as a bar to a subsequent suit.

Due Process: Requirement of the U.S. Constitution that all persons and business entities receive fair treatment in trials, hearings, and other legal, governmental, agency, or facility proceedings, and that legislation be fair to all.

Duty: An obligation recognized by the law. A health care provider's duty to a patient is to provide the degree of care ordinarily exercised by health care providers practicing under the same or similar circumstances in the same area of specialization.

Duty to Warn: Requirement that certain professions, generally in the behavioral health field, must warn an identifiable person of an express threat of violence made by a patient.

Economic Damages: All losses, including past and probable future medical expenses, loss of earnings and loss of future earnings (may take into consideration possible earnings from retirement accounts). Also includes loss of employment for business opportunities.

Emergency Medical Treatment and Active Labor Act (EMTALA): Federal legislation that requires a hospital to provide an appropriate medical screening examination to any person who comes to the hospital's emergency department and requests treatment or an examination for a medical condition, regardless of the individual's ability to pay. Applies to all hospitals that participate in the Medicare program and offer emergency services. It covers all patients, not just those who receive Medicare benefits.

Evidence: Facts presented at trial through witnesses, records, documents, objects, and other ways for the purpose of providing or defending a case. Some examples of evidence are as follows.

- *Circumstantial evidence:* facts or circumstances that indirectly imply that the principal facts at issue actually occurred.

- *Direct evidence:* proof of facts that establishes a fact directly without the necessity of the proof of any other fact.

- *Demonstrative/real evidence:* the use of articles or objects rather than the statement of witnesses to prove a fact in question.

- *Material evidence:* proof of facts that directly affects an element of the cause of action, such as standard of care testimony in a medical malpractice case.

- *Opinion evidence:* testimony of an expert witness based on special training or background, rather than on personal knowledge of the facts at issue.

- *Prima facie evidence:* a level of proof which is sufficient to establish the fact, and if not rebutted, becomes conclusive of the fact.

Expert Opinion: The testimony of a person who has special training, knowledge, skill or experience in an area relevant to resolution of the legal dispute.

Federal Court: Federal courts are another system of trial and appellate courts like state courts, which only accept certain types of cases. Malpractice cases generally are not filed in the federal courts unless a patient is from one state and the health care provider is from another state.

Felony: A crime of a serious nature punishable by imprisonment for a period of longer than one year.

Foreseeability: The requirement that the case must be judged on the unique facts as they were at the time of the occurrence; not in retrospect or with hindsight.

Fraud: An example of an intentional tort. This involves deliberately misleading a patient as to events involved in her/his care. For example, if a surgeon discovers that a foreign object has been left in the patient which needs to be removed, the surgeon has an obligation to disclose this to the patient.

Good Samaritan Law: Enacted by each state to provide limited protection for health care providers who stop at the scene of an accident or render medical assistance in an emergency.

Grand Jury: Group of citizens who are summoned and returned by the sheriff to each session of the criminal courts, and whose duty it is to receive complaints and accusations in criminal cases, hear the evidence adduced on the part of the state, and find bills of indictment in cases where they are satisfied a trial should be held. They are first sworn, and instructed by the court.

Group Health Plan ERISA: insured and self-insured plans that have 50 or more participants or is administered by an entity other than the employer.

Guardian Ad Litem: Guardian appointed by a court to act for one who is involved in a lawsuit and who cannot, for various reasons, legally act in his own behalf.

Hazardous Wastes: Wastes that contribute significantly to serious, irreversible illnesses or pose hazards to human health when improperly managed.

Health Care Clearinghouse: An entity that either:

- Processes or facilitates the processing of health information received from another entity in nonstandard format or containing nonstandard data content; or

- Receives a standard transaction from another entity and process or facilitates the processing of health information into nonstandard format or nonstandard data consent.

Health Care Quality Improvement Act (HCQIA): Federal legislation of 1986 that created the requirement for hospitals and State boards of medical examiners to report malpractice and incompetent performance to a national data bank; requires hospitals to query the national data bank prior to granting privileges to a physician; and provide incentive and protection to physicians engaging in effective professional peer review.

Health Care Provider: A provider of medical or health services or any other person or organization who furnishes, bills, or is paid for health care in the normal course of business.

Health Information: Any information, whether oral or recorded, that is created or received that relates to the past, present, or future physical or mental health of an individual or payment for health care.

Health Insurance Portability and Accountability Act (HIPAA): Federal legislation to protect health insurance coverage for workers and their families when they change or lose their jobs, national standards for electronic health care transactions, and requirements for the protection of the privacy of health information.

Health Plan: Individual or group that provides or pays the cost of health care.

Hearsay: Evidence not proceeding from the personal knowledge of the witness, but from the mere repetition of what he has heard others say. That which does not derive its value solely from the credit of the witness, but rests mainly on the veracity and competency of other persons. The very nature of the evidence shows its weakness, and it is admitted only in limited situations due to necessity.

Hung Jury: A jury that cannot come to a decision that constitutes a verdict in its jurisdiction, frequently after lengthy deliberation. A hung jury results in a mistrial, which in most circumstances means the case will be retried before a new jury.

Incident Report: Term for the report of a situation which is not consistent with the routine operation of a health care facility or the routine care of a particular patient. Incident reports are created in anticipation of potential litigation and are confidential.

Individual: A patient; member or client.

Individually Identifiable Health Information: Health information that identifies the individual or it's reasonably believed to be sufficient to identify the individual.

Informed Consent: The duty for giving information to a patient so an informed decision can be made regarding a procedure or treatment.

Injunction: A prohibitive writ issued by a court of equity against a defendant forbidding the latter to do some act which he is threatening or attempting to commit, or restraining him in the continuance thereof. A court may issue an injunction if defendant's conduct is injurious to the plaintiff, and not such as can be adequately redressed by an action at law with money damages.

Interrogatories: A discovery procedure in which one party submits a series of written questions to the opposing party who must answer in writing under oath within a certain period of time. The answers are admissible at trial under certain circumstances.

Judgment: The final entry in the record of a case, which is binding upon the parties unless overturned or modified on appeal. A judgment typically consists of a finding in favor of one or more of the parties and an assessment of damages and costs.

Jury Trial: A trial in which six or twelve registered voters are impaneled to hear the evidence, determine the facts, and render a verdict.

Law: Binding standards or guidelines for actions or behavior in a society.

Legal Precedent: Refers to a case furnishing an example for a similar case arising subsequently.

Liability: Being legally obligated or accountable.

- *Joint and Several Liability:* liability that may be shared either among two or more parties or to only one or a few select members of the group, at the adversary's discretion.

- *Vicarious Liability/Respondent Superior:* civil liability for the torts of others. Employers are vicariously liable for the negligent acts of their employees committed within the scope of their employment.

- *Personal Liability:* liability in which one is personally accountable, a wronged party can seek satisfaction out of the wrongdoer's personal assets.

Litigation: A lawsuit or legal action in court to determine legal issues, rights and duties between the parties to the litigation.

Loss of Consortium: A claim for damages by the spouse of an injured party for the loss of care, comfort, society, and interference with sexual relations.

Malpractice: Professional negligence. In medical terms, malpractice is the failure to exercise that degree of care as is used by reasonably prudent health care providers of like qualifications in the same or similar circumstances. The failure to meet this acceptable standard of care must cause or contribute to the patient injury to result in liability.

Minimum Necessary: When requesting, using, or disclosing PHI, an entity shall make reasonable efforts to limit PHI to the minimum necessary for the intended purpose of the use or disclosure. There are exceptions for: treatment; pursuant to an authorization, providing information to HHS; when required by law; and to comply with the HIPAA regulations.

Misdemeanor: An unlawful act of a less serious nature than a felony, usually punishable by fine or imprisonment for a term of less than a year.

Mistrial: An erroneous, invalid, or nugatory trial; a trial of an action which cannot stand in law because of want of jurisdiction, or a wrong drawing of jurors, or disregard of some other fundamental requisite.

Motion: Written or oral court plea requesting that a judge make an order or ruling affecting the lawsuit.

Negligence: Legal cause of action involving the failure to exercise the degree of diligence and care that a reasonably and ordinarily prudent person would exercise under the same or similar circumstances.

Non-Economic Damages: Compensation for non-monetary losses such as pain and suffering, emotional distress, loss of companionship, and loss of enjoyment of life.

Notary Public: A public official who administers oaths and certifies the validity of documents.

Occurrence Policy: Provides coverage even when the claim is filed after the policy is no longer in effect as long as the act of negligence occurred during the term of the insurance policy.

Opening Statement: Initial overview of a case that is given in a trial.

Patient Abandonment: Leaving a patient or assignment after accepting responsibility for patient care without first notifying the appropriate person to maintain the continuation of nursing care thereby endangering the health, safety and welfare of patients. State Boards of Nursing generally do not consider refusal to accept additional shifts or refusal to work overtime as patient abandonment.

Patient Record: The document containing pertinent health information concerning a patient. May also be referred to as a "medical record" or "clinical record."

Patient Self-Determination Act: Federal legislation that requires hospitals to inform all adult patients about their rights to accept or refuse medical or surgical treatment and the right to execute an advance directive.

Payment: The activities undertaken to obtain premiums or determine responsibility for coverage and the provision of health care benefits, or to obtain or provide reimbursement for health care services.

Plaintiff: The individual initiating the lawsuit. This may be the patient or the legal representative of the patient if the patient is a minor, incompetent, or deceased.

Pleading: First phase of a lawsuit, during which the issues in dispute are identified and clarified, including the plaintiff's cause of action and the defendant's grounds of defense.

Power of Attorney: Written instrument by which a person appoints another as his or her agent and confers on the other the authority to perform certain specified acts.

Precedent: A previous decision relied upon by a court for authority in making a current decision.

Pretrial Conference: Meeting held prior to trial at which an effort is made to resolve the issues still in dispute.

Privileged Communication: Confidential communication between individuals that attains a special legal status because of the nature of the individuals' relationship. The recipient of the communication can neither be legally compelled to disclose it as a witness nor voluntarily disclose it without the permission of the person making the disclosure. Privileged communications include communications such as between attorney and client, husband and wife, physician and patient, and priest and penitent.

Protected Heath Information (PHI): Individually identifiable health information that is transmitted or maintained in any form or medium.

Psychotherapy Notes: Notes recorded by a mental health professional documenting or analyzing the contents of conversions during a counseling session and that are maintained separately from the individual's medical record.

Punitive Damages: Additional damages awarded to punish the wrongdoer for willful misconduct; intended to punish the wrongdoer, not to compensate for the injured party's loss.

Respondeat Superior: "Let the master answer." The legal principle that makes an employer liable for civil wrongs committed by employees within the course and scope of their employment.

Respondent: Person who argues against a petition on appeal, generally the person who prevailed in the lower court.

Risk Management: A systems approach to the prevention of malpractice claims; involves identification of system problems as well as identification of patients who may sue. Process includes identification, analysis and treatment of risks.

Settlement: An agreement made between the parties to a lawsuit or a claim which resolves their legal dispute.

Small Claims Court: Special court that hears minor cases and uses simplified procedures.

Standard of Care: Norms of behavior and action as defined by a particular profession.

Statute of Limitations: The legislation which requires court cases to be filed within a limited period commencing with the date a wrong occurs or is (or should be) discovered.

Statutory Laws: Laws that have been formally adopted by legislative bodies.

Subpoena: Court order requiring a witness to appear before a court to give testimony.

Subpoena Duces Tecum: Court order requiring the production of documents in a legal proceeding.

Summary Health Information: Information that summarizes claims history, claims expenses, or type of claims for whom a plan sponsor has provided health benefits under a group health plan and the information has been de-identified.

Summary Judgment: Granting of a judgment in favor of either party prior to trial. Summary judgment is only granted when there is no factual dispute and one of the parties is entitled to judgment as a matter of law.

Summons: A court order directed to the sheriff to notify the defendant that an action has been filed against him or her and that he or she is required to appear, on a day named, and answer the complaint.

Tail Coverage: Special insurance coverage that can be purchased upon termination of a claims-made policy. Coverage extends to claims or suits filed after the expiration of a policy; called reporting endorsement coverage. Tail coverage is usually purchased when a person retires from practice, changes insurance coverage, or moves to another state where the existing coverage is unavailable.

Telemedicine: The practice of medicine by a physician located outside the state, treatment of a patient or rendering a medical opinion concerning the diagnosis of a patient by a physician in another state as a result of the transmission of individual patient data by electronic or other means. A method of health care service delivery used to facilitate medical consultations by physicians to health care providers in rural or underserved areas for the purpose of patient diagnosis or treatment that requires advanced telecommunications technologies including interactive video consultation, teleradiology and telepathology (TAC § 355.7001)(a)(1)). The practice of health care delivery, diagnosis, consultation, treatment, transfer of medical data, or exchange of medical education information by means of audio, video, or data communications. Telemedicine is not a consultation provided by telephone or facsimile machine. (36 Okl. Stat. § 6802).

Tort Law: Legal system's recognition of an injured party's right to seek compensatory damages for personal injuries.

Transaction: Transmission of information between two parties to carry out financial or administrative activities related to health care.

Treatment: The provision, coordination, or management of health care and related services by a health care provider or between health care providers and a third party or another health care provider.

Use: With respect to individually identifiable health information, the sharing, employment, application, utilization, examination, or analysis of such information.

Venue: The place or county in which an injury is declared to have been done, or fact declared to have happened. The county or district in which an action is brought for trial, and which is to furnish the panel of jurors.

Vicarious Liability/Respondeat Superior: Civil liability for the torts of others. Employers are vicariously liable for the negligent acts of their employees committed within the scope of their employment.

Wrongful Birth: An action brought by parents who seek damages after the birth of an unwanted or unplanned child. The parents assert that they received inadequate medical care that led to the birth of a child and that if they had received proper treatment, the child's birth could have been avoided.

Wrongful Death: An action at law, created by statute that permits the heirs and next of kin to recover money damages from the decedent's tortfeasor for the losses resulting from the decedent's death. The elements of the cause of action are established by statute in each state.

Wrongful Life: An action brought by an impaired child who contends that if his or her parents had been correctly counseled about likely birth defects, he or she never would have been conceived or would have been aborted.

STUDY PACKAGE
CONTINUING EDUCATION
CREDIT INFORMATION

LEGAL AND ETHICAL STANDARDS
FOR NURSES

Thank you for choosing PESI Healthcare as your continuing education provider. Our goal is to provide you with current, accurate and practical information from the most experienced and knowledgeable speakers and authors.

Listed below are the continuing education credit(s) currently available for this self-study package. **Please note, your state licensing board dictates whether self study is an acceptable form of continuing education. Please refer to your state rules and regulations.*

Nurses: PESI HealthCare, LLC, Eau Claire is an approved provider of continuing nursing education by the Wisconsin Nurses Association Continuing Education Approval Program Committee, an accredited approver by the American Nurses Credentialing Center's Commission on Accreditation. This approval is accepted and/or recognized by all state nurses associations that adhere to the ANA criteria for accreditation. This learner directed educational activity qualifies for 6.0 contact hours. PESI Healthcare certification: CA #06538.

Procedures: 1. Read book.
              2. Complete the post-test/evaluation form and mail it along with payment to the address on the form.

Your completed test/evaluation will be graded. If you receive a passing score (80% and above), you will be mailed a certificate of successful completion with earned continuing education credits. If you do not pass the post-test, you will be sent a letter indicating areas of deficiency, references to the appropriate sections of the manual for review and your post-test. The post-test must be resubmitted and receive a passing grade before credit can be awarded.

If you have any questions, please feel free to contact our customer service department at 1-800-843-7763.

PESI HealthCare, LLC
200 SPRING ST. STE B, P.O. BOX 100
EAU CLAIRE, WI 54702-1000

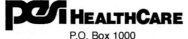

Legal and Ethical Standards
For Nurses

P.O. Box 1000
Eau Claire, WI 54702
(800) 843-7763

ZNT008780

This home study package includes CONTINUING
EDUCATION FOR ONE PERSON: complete and
return this original post/test evaluation form.

ADDITIONAL PERSONS interested in receiving
credit may photocopy this form, complete and
return with a payment of $25.00 per person CE fee.
A certificate of successful completion will be mailed
to you.

For office use only
Rcvd. _____
Graded _____
Cert. mld. _____

C.E. Fee: **$25**

Credit card # _____

Exp. Date _____

Signature _____

V-Code* _____ (***MC/VISA/Discover:** last 3-digit # on
signature panel on back of card.) (***American Express:** 4-digit # above
account # on face of card.)

**Mail to: PESI HealthCare, PO Box 1000, Eau Claire, WI 54702, or
Fax to: PESI HealthCare (800) 675-5026 (fax all pages)**

Name (please print): _____ _____ _____
                              LAST   FIRST   M.I.

Address: _____

City: _____ State: _____ Zip: _____

Daytime Phone: _____

Signature: _____

• Date you completed the PESI HC Tape/Manual Independent Package: _____

• Actual time (# of hours) taken to complete this offering: _____ hours

PROGRAM OBJECTIVES

How well did we do in achieving our seminar objectives?

	Excellent				Poor
Demonstrate understanding of the four elements of liability and how they are proven.	5	4	3	2	1
Explain the different types of professional liability insurance policies and the pros and cons of each.	5	4	3	2	1
Describe how a Nursing Regulatory Agency can take action against a nurse's license.	5	4	3	2	1
List key factors for effective depositions.	5	4	3	2	1
Describe circumstances in which health information may be used or disclosed without the patient's consent.	5	4	3	2	1
Explain the elements required for an informed decision.	5	4	3	2	1
Describe how treatment decisions may be made when a patient lacks capacity.	5	4	3	2	1

POST-TEST QUESTIONS

1. Identify the elements required for a jury to find a defendant liable in a malpractice action:

   a. captain of the ship; vicarious liability; delegation of a duty; harm to a patient

   b. damages; breach of the standard of care; injury or harm as a result of not meeting the standard of care; relationship between a nurse and the patient

   c. failure to follow a Policy; failure results in harm to a patient; the patient didn't trust the nurse; the nurse didn't like the patient

   d. personal accountability; corporate responsibility; delegation by a supervisor creating third-party liability; respondeat superior

2. A Nursing Regulatory Agency must allow a nurse an opportunity to meet with an investigator before a nursing license is suspended or terminated.

    ___ **True**   ___ **False**

3. Health information may be used or disclosed without a patient's consent under the following circumstances:

    a. a felony is committed by the patient

    b. the patient admits he abused his father

    c. the patient's cardiologist wants to consult about the patient with the patient's psychiatrist

    d. the health information is 20 years old

4. If a patient lacks capacity to make a treatment decision, the patient's spouse has the authority to make that treatment decision.

    ___ **True**   ___ **False**

5. The best type of professional liability insurance to purchase and the reason for that is:

    a. occurrence—coverage is available whenever the claim is brought, even after retirement from nursing

    b. claims-made—it is cheaper and covers a lawsuit whenever it is filed

    c. occurrence—tail coverage can be purchased at a lower cost

    d. claims-made—the American Nurses Association sells these types of policies

6. At trial, it is very important to be attentive to the proceedings, look at the jurors when testifying, and refer to the judge as "Your Honor."

    ___ **True**   ___ **False**

For additional forms and information on other PESI products, contact:
Customer Service; PESI HEALTHCARE;
P.O. Box 1000; Eau Claire, WI 54702
(Toll Free, 7 a.m.-5 p.m. central time, 800-843-7763).
www.pesihealthcare.com

Thank you for your comments.
We strive for excellence and we value your opinion.